How to Recover

from

Shoulder Surgery

How to Recover from Shoulder Surgery

Safe, Effective Recovery:

A Physiotherapist Shares 40 Years Experience Rehabilitating Shoulders

Bruce Paulik

Musculoskeletal Physiotherapist

BSc (Anatomy), BAppSc (Physiotherapy), GradDipMT

BTM Publishing

How to Recover from Shoulder Surgery
Safe, Effective Recovery: A Physiotherapist Shares 40
Years Experience Rehabilitating Shoulders
© Bruce Paulik 2020

Disclaimer

The medical and health information provided throughout this book is of a general nature and is provided as an educational resource. This general information about health conditions, surgery and treatment should not be used as an alternative to professional medical advice. This book does not address individual health circumstances, and so the relevance of the information provided should be confirmed by a qualified health professional such as a doctor, physiotherapist, nurse or pharmacist. The information is provided without any representations or warranties, expressed or implied. On this basis, the author and publishers disclaim all responsibilities for any loss, injury, claim, or damage of any kind resulting from the use of the information provided in this book.

Publisher
BTM Publishing, PO Box 248, Claremont WA 6910, Australia

ISBN: 978-0-6489127-1-2 (ebook)
ISBN: 978-0-6489127-0-5 (print)

NATIONAL LIBRARY OF AUSTRALIA

A catalogue record for this work is available from the National Library of Australia

Dedication

For my wife Tracey-Maree and son Michael,
who inspire me, and constantly encouraged
me to write this book.

About the Author

Bruce is an Australian Musculoskeletal Physio-therapist who has been in practice for over 40 years. His areas of special clinical interest include shoulder and neck pain, and orthopaedic shoulder rehabilitation.

Bruce started his special interest in shoulders during his studies at University—initially a Science Degree majoring in Anatomy, then his Physiotherapy Degree. This special interest continued during his postgraduate studies in Musculoskeletal Physiotherapy, and while teaching physiotherapy students.

He started in Private Practice in 1978, and by 1994 was also the Director of Physiotherapy Services at St John of God Hospital Murdoch. Over a 10-year period Bruce spent the majority of his clinical time working with the orthopaedic surgeons at Murdoch to provide shoulder rehabilitation programs.

He has always said that he is never happier than when working with patients to help them return to a full and active life. As a Musculoskeletal Physiotherapist Bruce has always felt like a clinical detective—watching for clues in a patient's story and their physical examination, and then coming to a diagnosis of a patient's pain or dysfunction. He sees that return to normal and pain free function is a partnership between the therapist and patient, with his role as both treating therapist and educator/coach.

Bruce has taught physiotherapy students and

lectured to medical practitioners about shoulder rehabilitation. He has been involved in clinical research in his area of special expertise—the management and treatment of shoulder problems. He has also served on various state and national committees of the Australian Physiotherapy Association.

Bruce is in practice at HFRC, a clinic in Nedlands, Western Australia, and consults there and online through telehealth video consultations. Go to www.hfrc.com.au

Acknowledgements

Thank you to all my patients, from whom I have learnt the lessons that I have included in this book.

I am grateful to all the physiotherapists and medical practitioners who, over the past 40 years, have taught, mentored, lectured and shared with me the wisdom of their knowledge and experience of treating shoulders.

Healing...

Healing is a matter of time, but it is
sometimes also a matter of opportunity.

– Hippocrates, the "Father of Medicine"

Physiotherapist or Physical Therapist

Throughout this book I will use the titles "Physiotherapist" and "Physical Therapist" interchangeably.

In the US the term Physical Therapist is widely used, although the use of Physiotherapist is becoming more common.

In most other countries Physiotherapist is used.

Table of Contents

Chapter 1

A Tale of Two Shoulders

L et me tell you the story of two patients with the same surgery on the same day who ultimately had very different recovery paths.

It was 1997. The young orthopaedic surgeons in the medical centre where my clinic was located were well-trained and using the latest techniques in shoulder surgery. On a Wednesday in mid-July two men presented for their first rehabilitation session 5 days after rotator cuff shoulder surgery—let's call them Bill and Jim.

Jim was 39 years old, fairly fit, but irritated that this process was taking him away from his work. He had had a moderate size rotator cuff tear repaired. Bill was 82 years old, fit and keen to get on with his rehabilitation. He also had a moderately sized rotator cuff tear repaired by the same surgeon with the same technique on the same day. At this point most clinicians would expect that Jim, being 40 years younger, would make a faster recovery than Bill. This was not to be the case.

Jim had done no preparation for his surgery. He was unaware of the details of his shoulder surgery and had read none of the printed materials supplied by the surgeon. He had not taken the surgeon's advice to see me for an exercise program prior to the surgery. Since the operation he was struggling at home with simple daily activities such as washing and dressing.

Bill, on the other hand, was well prepared for the surgery. He had in fact been to see me three weeks earlier and started a simple exercise program. He had read everything he could lay his hands on, so knew the post-operative process and how to manage at home, despite living alone.

From this point on, the differences between Jim and Bill increased further. Jim often missed review sessions with me, and at these sessions admitted to going at times several days without doing his simple home exercise program. His unspoken attitude was that if the surgeon had done an expert job, he shouldn't need to do any more. In contrast, Bill kept appointments, did a few minutes of exercise every day as instructed, but was careful not to over-stress the shoulder, and so protecting the repairing rotator cuff from injury.

And so how did Jim and Bill progress in their recovery? It would be great if I could say that with an excellent orthopaedic surgeon and the latest modern surgical techniques that they both had the same progress! Obviously this wasn't the case, otherwise I wouldn't be telling the story, I wouldn't need to write this book, and you wouldn't need to read it.

Bill's progress was better than average—his pain settled quickly in the postoperative period. By the time the surgeon allowed him to stop using the sling 5 weeks after surgery, his range of shoulder movement was improving rapidly. Importantly, he had coped well at home with his arm in a sling for 5 weeks. At 3 months he had almost full range of movement; by 6 months he was doing a "return to golf" rehabilitation exercise program.

Jim however was struggling. He refused to take the pain and anti-inflammatory medication that had been prescribed by his orthopaedic surgeon, and so his pain levels were much higher than Bill's. As he was only occasionally doing his home exercise program, and was experiencing significant pain, his shoulder was getting very stiff. He was taking advice from acquaintances rather than his health professionals, and so was attempting to overcome the stiffness by doing his exercises more aggressively but infrequently.

At five weeks when he was advised to stop wearing his sling, he experienced a spike in his pain level. At this point he had very poor active range of motion with marked pain at the limit of movement.

By six months after surgery Jim was still experiencing quite a lot of discomfort over the shoulder and could not sleep on that side. His active range of movement was still restricted in every direction.

At 12 months post-operatively he still had not reached the level of recovery that Bill had at six months.

Why I Was Driven To Write This Book

Cases like Bill and Jim, and countless others in the

20 years since then, have made me realise that it is the patient who controls their recovery, not me as their physical therapist.

Several years ago, as a guest of that same orthopaedic surgeon who operated on Bill and Jim, I attended a conference for orthopaedic surgeons who specialise in the shoulder. On the last day of the conference, at a panel discussion in front of the 450 delegates, a professor of orthopaedic surgery from the UK said

> *"Your orthopaedic surgery of the shoulder is only as good as the post-operative physiotherapy program."*

I would take that one step further and say:

> *"The post-operative recovery from orthopaedic surgery of the shoulder is only as good as the patient makes it."*

When I can help patients make the right decisions about their shoulder rehabilitation, and provide them with the knowledge and tools to have a speedy and effective recovery, then I am a happy Physiotherapist!

As I have publicly stated on LinkedIn:

> *"My purpose is to make a significant positive impact on the physical health of the clients who attend my physiotherapy clinic or consult with me online."*

This book allows me to do this on a grander scale, reaching far more people than I could in several lifetimes individually. I won't now be so frustrated by those who refuse to be helped. And so, I set out to make a positive and meaningful difference in the world with my words. And this book helps me reach more people and achieve that mission.

To take control of your recovery from shoulder surgery, you need to understand the basics of your surgery rehabilitation, and the process of healing. This will help you lose your anxiety and focus your attention and energies on getting well fast and efficiently. Recovery from shoulder surgery is a process, and it takes time. This timeline can be accelerated by avoiding complications, appreciating your physical limitations through each phase of the recovery process, and following the right steps in the process to promote faster healing.

Why You Should Read This Book

So who could benefit from reading this book?

This book will help if you or a loved one:

- ◆ Have been referred to an orthopaedic surgeon with a view to surgery for a shoulder problem.

- ◆ Have already seen an orthopaedic surgeon and are considering shoulder surgery based on the surgeon's advice.

- ◆ Have booked in for shoulder surgery.

- ◆ Have recently had shoulder surgery.

5

Once you understand the basics of the preparation for surgery, the surgery itself, and the rehabilitation program, there is much less fear and anxiety about the whole process. The predictability of the process becomes reassuring, allowing you to focus your entire attention and energy on rehabilitating your shoulder back to full pain-free function.

I hope the knowledge and tools in this book help you make a speedy recovery, with less anxiety and pain, and ultimately a better return to full function of your shoulder.

Chapter 2

A User's Guide to the Shoulder

The shoulder is easily the most amazing joint in the human body. If you don't believe me, watch international level gymnastics sometime and take notice of the incredible things that athletes do with their shoulders.

The shoulder has the largest range of movement of any joint in the body, and yet with the right training and fitness people can walk on their hands or carry out amazing manoeuvres on Roman rings at gymnastic competitions.

Analysing these abilities of the shoulder, we can see that the shoulder has mobility, strength and stability. These three are often seen as being mutually exclusive, but the shoulder manages all three in its optimum state.

So how does the shoulder girdle manage this? Because it comprises a complex of joints which are stabilised by a complex arrangement of muscles and ligaments:

◆ The glenohumeral joint (GHJ) is the "ball and socket" joint between the humerus (upper arm bone) and the scapula (shoulder blade). The socket is deepened by a ring of cartilage—the glenoid labrum. The glenoid labrum provides better stability.

- The acromioclavicular joint (ACJ) is the joint between the acromion (part of the scapula) and the clavicle (collar bone).

- The scapulothoracic articulation is not actually a joint but an area where the scapula moves across the ribs under the control of several muscles.

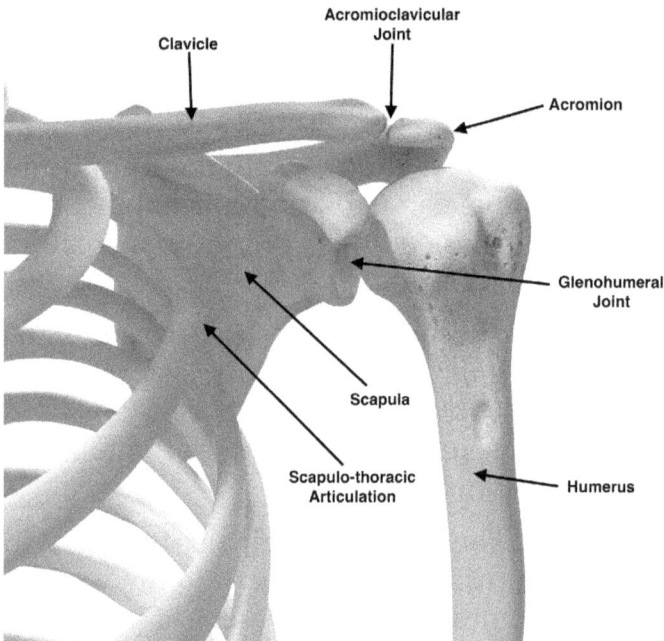

These joints are moved by and stabilised by a range of muscles. The most important group of muscles for the GHJ is the Rotator Cuff—the Supraspinatus, Infraspinatus, Subscapularis and Teres Minor muscles. These muscles attach the scapula to the head of the humerus and stabilise the GHJ. Their tendons form a cuff around the head of the humerus, providing both movement and stability.

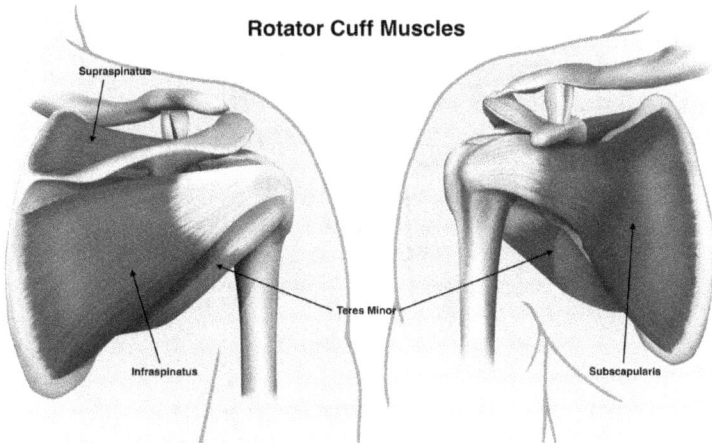

Rotator Cuff Muscles

Supraspinatus

Teres Minor

Infraspinatus

Subscapularis

Without a functioning rotator cuff, we are actually unable to raise our arm past horizontal. At the very least we experience shoulder pain on overhead activities, as the humeral head can rise compressing the subacromial/subdeltoid bursa. Damage to the rotator cuff is one of the most common reasons for shoulder surgery.

The GHJ is surrounded by a joint capsule, a sleeve of ligamentous type tissue strengthened by several ligaments. A potential complication of shoulder surgery is "frozen shoulder", where the capsule becomes inflamed and ultimately thickened and tight. This can cause restricted and painful movement and delayed recovery.

Shoulder Joint

Clavicle

Supraspinatus Muscle

Glenoid Labrum

Glenoid Cavity
Scapula

Articular Cartilage

Synovial Membrane
Fibrous Membrane

Articular Capsule

Acromioclavicular Ligament
Coracoacromial Ligament
Acromion of Scapula
Subacromial Bursa

Articular Capsule

Tendon Sheath
Head of Humerus

Humerus

Biceps Brachii Muscle

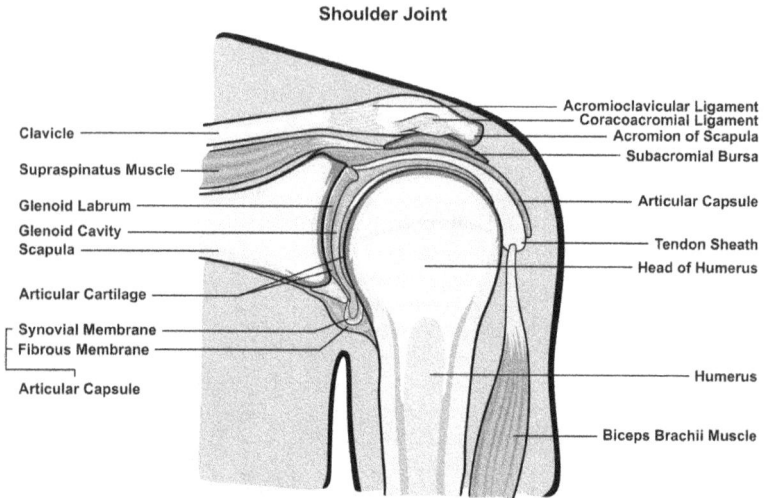

So in summary the glenohumeral joint:

◆ is a large ball sitting in a small shallow socket,

◆ is held together by a loose joint capsule (to allow a large range of movement),

◆ has a capsule strengthened by several ligaments,

◆ is stabilised by the rotator cuff group of muscles and their tendons, and

◆ is moved by many muscles travelling between the spine, thorax, scapula and upper arm.

In this way the shoulder meets our requirements of mobility, stability and strength. It does however leave the shoulder susceptible to any injury or degenerative changes of these structures.

Although a rehabilitation exercise program can achieve a lot, there will be times where surgical help is required.

If you want to see how all these structures move together, I suggest a Shoulder Anatomy Animated Tutorial narrated by an orthopaedic surgeon, and other shoulder anatomy resources at:

www.theshoulderphysio.com/anatomy.

Chapter 3

Do I Really Need Surgery?

We can see from the anatomy of the region that to maintain a normal pain free shoulder, we need the health of a wide range of structures in the shoulder complex.

These structures–muscles, tendons, ligaments–can be affected by acute injury, chronic stress, repetitive injury, or degenerative changes over time.

The following list includes the most common shoulder problems that may require surgery.

Bursitis & Tendonitis

If the subacromial bursa or the rotator cuff tendons are subjected to pinching or rubbing under the acromion by repetitive activities, then they can become swollen, inflamed and painful. These problems by themselves should not need surgery if you have seen a competent physiotherapist to rehabilitate your shoulder.

With the correct rehabilitation program, many of the causes of bursitis or tendonitis can be eliminated by:

◆ altering your activities (whether work, sport or leisure),

◆ specific exercises to stretch or strengthen, and

◆ ice packs, medication or injections to settle inflammation.

Impingement & Partial Rotator Cuff Tears

Acute injury, repeated minor injuries or chronic physical stress from work, sport or normal daily activities can cause impingement of the rotator cuff tendons under the acromion. This can lead to a partial thickness tear of a rotator cuff tendon, where the tendon is damaged but not completely severed.

These tears may be associated with chronic inflammation of the tendon and bursa, and over time bony spurs can develop on the underside of the acromion. This may lead to further pressure and irritation of the tendon and bursa, with progression of the tears.

The spurs can be removed by arthroscopic surgery, at which time the tendon can be repaired if necessary. The presence of spurs increases the likelihood that surgery will be required, and a conservative rehab program by itself may not be sufficient to return your shoulder to normal pain free function.

Full-Thickness Rotator Cuff Tears

The rotator cuff may already be partially torn or weakened—typically in the middle-aged and older patient. Further injury or over-stress can lead to a full-thickness tear of one or more of the rotator cuff tendons. In this case, the tearing of the tendon leaves a gap between the tendon and the humeral head of the shoulder. As with impingement/partial tears,

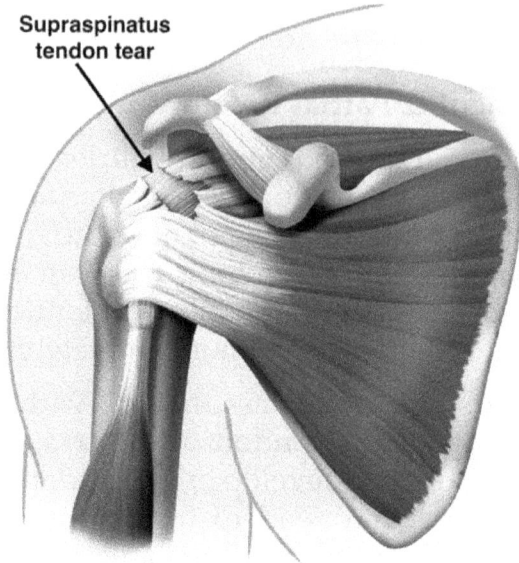

Supraspinatus
tendon tear

conservative nonsurgical management (such as activity modification, exercise rehabilitation and treatment of the inflammation) can be successful in returning the shoulder to normal function.

Often the extent of the damage is too great and surgical repair is required. If you have been doing a rehab exercise program for over 3 months under the supervision of a competent physiotherapist without substantial improvement, then it's time to see an orthopaedic surgeon for an opinion on surgery.

With these 3 categories, it may take 3 to 6 months to rehabilitate your shoulder fully without surgery. But don't be misled into thinking that it's Rehab OR Surgery—the choice is Rehab OR Surgery **plus** Rehab!

Instability

Instability of the shoulder means that the shoulder is too loose and can slide around too easily in its socket. A *subluxation* occurs when the ball rides up onto the edge of the socket on the glenoid labrum, but then slips back into place. If the ball comes completely out of the socket, it is a *dislocation*. This instability can result from injury such as a forceful dislocation playing sport, or due to a generalised laxity of the ligaments of the body—so called "double jointed" people.

A complete dislocation can damage tissues around the shoulder, predisposing to further instability and increased chance of further dislocations. Damage to the glenoid labrum with subluxation or dislocation can cause pain, further instability and a loss of strength. A specific rehab exercise program can strengthen the stabilising muscles around the shoulder. If the shoulder stabilising structures (the joint capsule and ligaments) are too loose, you may find that the benefit from the exercises is not enough to allow you to return to your normal activities. There are "key hole" surgery techniques that will tighten the shoulder structures.

Arthritis

Osteoarthritis and rheumatoid arthritis can lead to a gradual wearing away of the articular cartilage lining the ball and the socket. Furthermore, there can be degeneration and tearing of the rotator cuff, and deterioration of the joint capsule. Over time these changes will cause increasing pain with decreased range of movement and shoulder strength. With mild to moderate degenerative changes, an exercise program to maintain strength and range of movement can give you a pain free shoulder with adequate function. With more advanced degeneration of the shoulder where exercising is not sufficient, surgical options include a hemiarthroplasty where the humeral head alone is replaced, or total shoulder arthroplasty where both the ball and socket are replaced.

So what are your options?

Option 1

After appropriate imaging (Xray, ultrasound, MRI) you are assessed by a physical therapist with special expertise in shoulder rehab for an exercise rehabilitation program. Your medical practitioner may have prescribed medication or injections to help settle inflammation. If this achieves some improvement after 6 weeks, you continue this program of daily exercises, with the program being progressed at regular intervals by your physical therapist. After 3 to 6 months you achieve full shoulder function without pain. No surgery required!

Option 2

You have been doing your rehab exercises regularly as directed by your physical therapist for at least 6 weeks, but there are no signs of improvement, or improvement has reached a plateau. You discuss your progress with your physical therapist and medical practitioner and are referred to an orthopaedic surgeon for an opinion. The surgeon will recommend either continuing with rehab longer or progressing on to immediate surgery.

Option 3

Because your symptoms are severe, or due to the nature of the damage/degeneration seen on imaging, you are referred directly to an orthopaedic surgeon by your medical practitioner. Ask the surgeon about the pros and cons of a rehab exercise program versus surgery. Reputable surgeons work closely with physical therapists who have special expertise with the shoulder and won't hesitate to refer you if they can see benefit from a trial of conservative care with a rehab exercise program.

It is becoming much more common now for patients to be referred for an exercise program prior to surgery to help improve pain, range of movement and strength (see the chapter "Prehab before Rehab").

A second opinion?

If, having seen an orthopaedic surgeon who has suggested surgery, you are still undecided about going ahead, speak to your medical practitioner about a referral to another orthopaedic surgeon for a second opinion. This is perfectly acceptable—after all it is *your* body and *your* health—you need to be assured that going ahead to surgery is the right decision. When you are confident that it is the right decision, then you are in the right frame of mind for the best recovery from the surgery.

Chapter 4

Common Types of Surgery and What to Expect

Arthroscopic Acromioplasty/Subacromial Decompression

Arthroscopic acromioplasty and subacromial decompression/debridement/smoothing is an arthroscopic (keyhole surgery) procedure to provide more space for the bursa and tendons - it is used to treat impingement and bursitis of the shoulder.

The procedure involves inserting a pencil like camera through one or more small incisions over the shoulder. This allows the surgeon to view both the shoulder joint and the subacromial space, where the area of bursitis and impingement can be viewed directly. The subacromial smoothing shaves bone from the underneath of the acromion process. This results in increased subacromial space and decreased pressure and irritation of the tendons and bursa. Inflamed and swollen bursa or damaged tendon material may also be trimmed away during the procedure.

You may have a general anaesthetic during this procedure, or a regional nerve block (or perhaps both). A regional nerve block involves an injection into the side of the base of the neck, leaving the shoulder & arm numb for 12 to 24 hours. The most common type for shoulder surgery is the Interscalene Block.

A rehabilitation exercise program is vital to regain range of movement, strength and function of the shoulder after arthroscopic surgery. Although you will initially wear a sling for comfort, you will do some gentle range of motion exercises in the first few days.

The rehabilitation program will gradually progress to more strengthening and joint control type exercises. Average recovery times are given below, but individuals will progress at different rates depending on their age, associated injuries, pre-injury health status, compliance with the rehabilitation exercise program and injury severity.

Expected recovery process & timeline

(How long will my recovery take, and what will I be doing during my recovery?)

◆ It's common to go home the same day (day surgery), but you may remain in hospital until the next day after the surgery. The surgeon will determine when you're ready to return home.

◆ Your physical therapist will show you gentle exercises to begin immediately at home. These exercises are important - they start the process of maintaining and then improving your mobility and muscle strength.

◆ During the first three weeks you should continue to do your home exercise program 3 times daily. These are gentle exercises and should be carried out exactly to the physical therapist's instructions. (See Chapter 13 for examples of these early exercises.)

◆ By 6 weeks you will be experiencing minimal pain and notice steadily improving active range of movement. You will be gradually returning to your normal activities.

◆ By 12 to 16 weeks you will be making a gradual return to sport and work activities, including those that require overhead movements such as throwing, swimming, racquet sports.

Functional limitations during recovery

(What can I do and not do during my recovery?)

◆ There are no particular restrictions placed on shoulder movement. In fact, you will be best served by moving the arm in your daily activities within the painfree range of movement.

◆ You will be wearing a sling for comfort for 2 weeks, but pain permitting you can do without the sling earlier. It's worth remembering when going out into social situations or crowded areas that the sling acts as a warning to others that you have an injured arm!

◆ You may not drive while you remain in the sling.

◆ It's common to feel pain during activity and even at rest during the first three weeks.

◆ During the first 3 weeks you should avoid activities that put pressure on the area of bone under the acromion that has been shaved down.

Expected final outcome

(How good will my shoulder be at the end of the rehabilitation time?)

◆ By 4 to 6 months the shoulder should be pain free, with full range of motion and normal strength.

◆ By 12 months function of the shoulder in activities of daily living, sport and work should be normal. This outcome depends on an appropriate rehabilitation exercise program, performed conscientiously and sensibly.

Arthroscopic Labrum Repair & Shoulder Stabilization

The shoulder joint is a very shallow ball and socket joint, allowing great freedom of movement, but leaving the shoulder with less stability. The glenoid labrum is the ring of fibrous cartilage that deepens the shoulder socket, contributing to better stability. Injuries such as a fall onto an outstretched hand or a shoulder dislocation can damage the labrum, even tearing a portion away from the bone. The most common labrum damage requiring surgery is the SLAP (Superior Labral Anterior Posterior) tear, which is usually repaired arthroscopically using sutures and small bone anchors. You will probably go home the same day, with your arm in a sling for 3 to 6 weeks, depending on the extent of the repair.

Shoulder Instability implies that your shoulder can dislocate or sublux easily during activity. Subluxation means that the shoulder ball moves further than it should in the socket, but doesn't completely dislocate, before returning to a normal position. Shoulder dislocation or subluxation can result from trauma, causing damage to the labrum or joint capsule, which may require surgical repair.

Atraumatic dislocation or subluxation can result from muscle imbalances & weakness around the shoulder, or be due to inherent laxity of the supporting structures of the shoulder, for instance in people with general joint laxity.

In either case, the first approach is a comprehensive rehabilitation exercise program designed by a physiotherapist with expertise in this area. If this approach is ultimately unsuccessful, then surgery to repair labral damage or tighten the joint capsule may be required.

Expected recovery process & timeline

(How long will my recovery take, and what will I be doing during my recovery?)

- ◆ It's quite common to go home the same day (day surgery), but you may remain in hospital until the next day after the surgery, with the surgeon determining when you're ready to return home.

◆ Your physical therapist will show you gentle exercises to begin immediately at home. These exercises will maintain elbow and hand function, but not move the shoulder joint. You may also be doing gentle exercise for the muscles around the shoulder blade (scapula).

◆ During the first 4 weeks you should continue to do your home exercise program 3 times daily. These are gentle exercises, and should be carried out exactly to the physical therapist's instructions (see Chapter 13 for examples of these early exercises).

◆ By 6 weeks you will be experiencing minimal pain and notice steadily improving active range of movement. You will be gradually returning to your normal activities.

◆ By 12 to 16 weeks you will be making a gradual return to sport and work activities, including those that require overhead movements such as throwing, swimming, racquet sports.

Functional limitations during recovery

(What can I do and not do during my recovery?)

◆ The surgeon will place particular restrictions on shoulder movement, depending on the structures damaged & repaired during surgery. You will not be allowed to move the shoulder actively during the first 4 weeks, being restricted to gentle passive movement eg: when you allow the arm to hang down (see Chapter 13 for these exercises), or movement by your physical therapist.

◆ You will be wearing a sling for about 4 weeks, 24 hours per day except when showering or doing exercises.

◆ You will not be allowed to drive while you remain in the sling.

◆ It's common to feel pain during activity and even at rest during the first three weeks.

◆ You will start exercises to regain movement and strength from about 5 weeks.

◆ By 12 weeks you will be starting sports specific rehabilitation.

◆ Return to work:
  • Office duties - 2 weeks, depending on pain.
  • Light manual duties - 8 weeks.
  • Heavy manual duties - 3 months

◆ Return to sport:
  • Fitness training - 6 weeks
  • Non-contact sports (no throwing) & swimming - 3 months
  • Light throwing (progressive program) - 4 to 5 months

- Gradual return to full overhead & contact sports - 6 months onwards.

Expected final outcome

(How good will my shoulder be at the end of the rehabilitation time?)

◆ By 4 to 6 months the shoulder should be pain free, with full range of motion and normal strength.

◆ By 12 months function of the shoulder in activities of daily living, sport and work should be normal. However, exercises such as bench press, inclined press or push-ups where the elbows move behind the line of the body are likely to over stretch the structures repaired, and result in further shoulder dislocation.

Acromioclavicular Joint Stabilization

Acromioclavicular joint injuries are a common occurrence in contact sports such as rugby and football, with the mechanism of injury being either a direct fall onto the tip of the shoulder or an indirect strain through the outstretched arm.

The extent of the injury will depend on which ligaments are damaged, and the severity of the damage. Commonly injuries to the AC joint are classified as Type I, Type II or Type III. Injuries classify as Type I or II will normally do well with a physical therapy rehabilitation program. In Type III injuries there is extensive damage with complete rupture of the coracoclavicular ligaments. This will result in dislocation and separation of the acromion and clavicle.

While some patients with a type III injury will give a satisfactory result from a rehabilitation program, the younger more athletic patient may require surgery to stabilise the joint. There are a variety of surgical procedures for AC joint stabilisation, and most will require immobilising the shoulder and arm in a sling for at least four weeks, followed by a graduated rehabilitation program.

Every patient will have their own unique post-operation experience depending on the surgical procedure used, and you will need to check with your surgeon. We can give some guidelines for your recovery:

Expected recovery process & timeline

(How long will my recovery take, and what will I be doing during my recovery?)

- It's common to go home the same day (day surgery), but you may remain in hospital until the next day after the surgery, with the surgeon determining when you're ready to return home.

- Your physical therapist will show you gentle exercises to begin immediately at home. These exercises will maintain elbow and hand function, but not move the shoulder joint. You may also be doing gentle exercises for the muscles around the shoulder blade (scapula).

◆ During the first 4 weeks you should continue to do your home exercise program 3 times daily. These are gentle exercises, and you should perform them exactly to the physical therapist's instructions (see Chapter 13 for examples of these early exercises).

◆ By 6 weeks you will be experiencing minimal pain and notice steadily improving active range of movement. You will be gradually returning to your normal activities.

◆ By 12 to 16 weeks you will be making a gradual return to sport and work activities, excluding those that require overhead movements such as throwing, swimming, racquet sports.

Functional limitations during recovery

(What can I do and not do during my recovery?)

◆ The surgeon will place particular restrictions on shoulder movement, depending on the surgical procedure used. You will not be allowed to move the shoulder actively during the first 4 weeks, being restricted to gentle passive movement eg: when you allow the arm to hang down (see Chapter 13 for these exercises), or movement by your physical therapist.

◆ You will wear a sling for about 4 weeks, 24 hours per day unless showering or doing exercises.

- You will not be allowed to drive while you remain in the sling.

- It's common to feel pain during activity and even at rest during the first three weeks.

- You will start exercises to regain movement and strength from about 5 weeks.

- By 12 weeks you will be starting sports specific rehabilitation.

- Return to work:
  - Office duties - 2 weeks, depending on pain.
  - Light manual duties - 12 weeks.
  - Heavy manual duties - 4 to 6 months

- Return to sport:
  - Fitness training - 6 weeks
  - Non-contact sports (no throwing) & swimming - 3 months
  - Light throwing (progressive program) - 4 to 5 months
  - Gradual return to full overhead & contact sports - 6 months onwards.

Expected final outcome

(How good will my shoulder be at the end of the rehabilitation time?)

- By 4 to 6 months the shoulder should be pain

free, with full range of motion and normal strength.

◆ By 12 months function of the shoulder in activities of daily living, sport and work should be normal. However, exercises such as bench press, inclined press or push-ups where the elbows move behind the line of the body are likely to over-stretch the structures repaired, and result in further AC joint instability.

Rotator Cuff Repair

Patients with full-thickness tears of one or more rotator cuff tendons will often not do well with a conservative rehabilitation program, and will require surgical repair of the tears. The repair is performed either arthroscopically, or with a small incision over the tip of the shoulder (a "mini-open" repair) for larger rotator cuff tears. The surgery is usually performed using a combination of general anaesthetic and local arm anaesthetic block which numbs the affected shoulder and arm for 12 to 24 hours. Small anchors with thread attached are placed in the bone, and the healthy rotator cuff tissue is tied back down to the bone.

You will return home after surgery on the same or next day, and need to wear a supporting sling for the next 4 to 6 weeks. The sling may incorporate a small pillow to keep the arm slightly away from the side, and although you'll have exercises to perform, you will not be allowed to lift the arm actively against gravity for 4 to 6 weeks.

While every patient will have their own unique post-operation experience, we can give some guidelines for your recovery:

Expected recovery process & timeline

(How long will my recovery take, and what will I be doing during my recovery?)

◆ It's quite common to go home the same day (day surgery), but usually you will remain in hospital until the next day after the surgery, with the surgeon determining when you're ready to return home. You will need to wear a supporting sling for the next 4 to 6 weeks.

◆ Your physical therapist will show you gentle exercises to begin immediately at home during the period that you are wearing the sling. These exercises are important–they start the process of maintaining and then improving your mobility and muscle strength. Without these early exercises your shoulder will become very stiff, leading to increased pain. With increased stiffness and pain there would be further inhibition of muscle activity around your shoulder, and the muscles will become even weaker, making your recovery slower when you stop wearing the sling.

◆ It's important to realize that the tendons are very slow to heal - this healing may not be complete for up to 6 months. The exact timing of your rehabilitation program will depend on the quality of the tendons repaired, and the size of the tear, so you must listen to your surgeon and physical therapist for guidance.

◆ During the first six weeks you should continue to do your home exercise program 2 to 3 times daily. These are very gentle exercises, and should be carried out exactly to the physical therapist's instructions. (See Chapter 13 for examples of these early exercises.)

◆ Once the sling is removed, you will move onto a more active exercise program under your physical therapist's guidance, to build better strength and mobility.

◆ By 3 months you will be experiencing minimal pain and notice steadily improving active range of movement. You will be gradually returning to your normal activities.

Functional limitations during recovery

(What can I do and not do during my recovery?)

◆ Your arm will remain in a sling for up to 6 weeks.

◆ You will not be allowed to drive while you remain in the sling.

◆ You will not be allowed to raise the arm actively from the sling. All movements of the shoulder will be done *passively*, either by the other hand, by gravity, or by your physical therapist.

◆ It's common to feel pain during activity and even at rest during the first six weeks.

◆ Initially you will have trouble with many of the normal activities of daily living, such as getting dressed, doing the laundry, showering, and preparing food. It is best to arrange help at home for at least the first 1 to 2 weeks.

Expected final outcome

(How good will my shoulder be at the end of the rehabilitation time?)

◆ By 3 to 6 months most patients are essentially pain-free (although cold weather may still make the shoulder ache - use a hot pack!). At 1 year post-op you will have achieved most of your functional recovery, with discomfort, range of movement and strength continuing to improve during this time.

◆ By 6 months after surgery you should be able to return to activities that are non-contact and low load eg golf, cycling, swimming. Activities involving repeated over head movements will take longer (eg tennis), as will contact and high impact sports. My advice - allow 12 months to return to full function.

◆ If you had a very large rotator cuff tear, and the surgeon indicates that the tendon was not of good quality, it possible that the repair will not hold in the longer term. This does not necessarily mean that you will have a poor outcome - many patients have a very functional shoulder, although with some overhead weakness if this happens.

Total Shoulder Replacement

Total Shoulder Replacement (TSR) is usually needed for shoulders with severe arthritis or bony injury. Arthritis causes wearing away of the cartilage that lines the surface of the bones in the joint leading to stiffness, inflammation and pain. When the symptoms are limiting your lifestyle, with constant pain and poor sleep at night, it is time to consider a TSR.

Types of TSR:

Hemi-arthroplasty

In this case only the humeral head needs to be replaced due to arthritis or injury. This avoids the risk of the glenoid component loosening later, and is an option for the younger more active patient. Should the glenoid socket become worn later, then further surgery may be required to convert this to a full replacement of the shoulder joint.

Total shoulder arthroplasty

Where both the ball (humeral head) and the glenoid socket are damaged:

◆ from injury or

◆ due to loss of the articular cartilage lining the surface of the bones because of arthritis, then a total shoulder replacement is called for, and both the humeral head and the socket are replaced by a combination of metal and/or plastic inserts. The obvious advantage over a hemi-arthroplasty is that further surgery shouldn't be required due to further deterioration of the glenoid socket from arthritis.

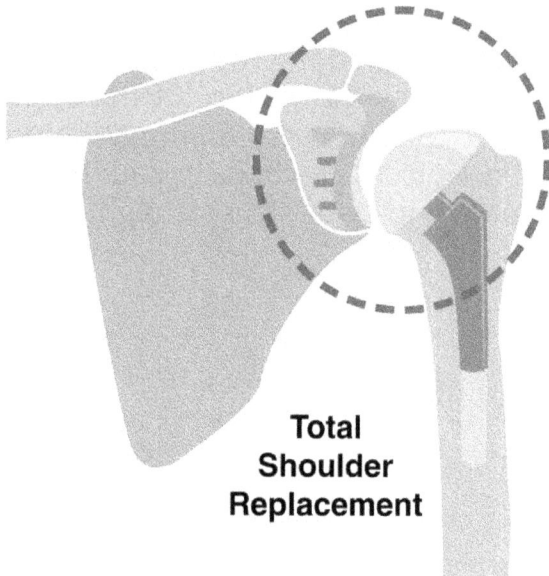

Total Shoulder Replacement

Reverse total shoulder replacement

If the rotator cuff is completely torn and cannot be repaired, then the results from a standard total shoulder arthroplasty are unlikely to be satisfactory. A reverse total shoulder replacement does not depend on an intact rotator cuff to give good pain-free function for the shoulder. In this procedure the ball and socket inserts are reversed, so that the socket is at the top of the humerus and the ball is attached where the socket had previously existed.

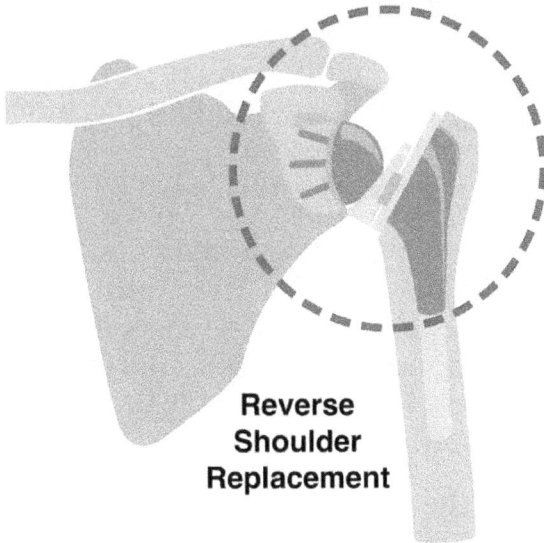

**Reverse
Shoulder
Replacement**

While every patient will have their own unique post-operation experience, we can give some guidelines for your recovery:

Expected recovery process & timeline

(How long will my recovery take, and what will I be doing during my recovery?)

- ◆ You will remain in hospital for a day or two after the surgery, with the surgeon determining when you're ready to return home.

- ◆ Your physical therapist will show you gentle exercises to begin immediately at home. These exercises are important–they start the process of maintaining and then improving your mobility and muscle strength. Without these early exercises your shoulder will

35

become very stiff, leading to increased pain. With increased stiffness and pain there would be further inhibition of muscle activity around your shoulder, and the muscles will become even weaker.

◆ During the first six weeks you should continue to do your home exercise program 2 to 3 times daily. These are very gentle exercises, and should be carried out exactly to the physical therapist's instructions. (See Chapter 13 for examples of these early exercises.)

◆ Once the sling is removed, you will move onto a more active exercise program under your physical therapist's guidance, to build better strength and mobility.

◆ By 3 months you will be experiencing minimal pain and notice steadily improving active range of movement. You will be gradually returning to your normal activities.

Functional limitations during recovery

(What can I do and not do during my recovery?)

◆ Your arm will remain in a sling for up to 6 weeks.

◆ You will not be allowed to drive while you remain in the sling.

◆ It's common to feel pain during activity and even at rest during the first six weeks.

◆ Initially you will have trouble with many of the normal activities of daily living, such as getting dressed, doing the laundry, showering, and preparing food. It is best to arrange help at home for at least the first 1 to 2 weeks.

Expected final outcome

(How good will my shoulder be at the end of the rehabilitation time?)

◆ By 6 months to one year most patients are essentially pain free (although cold weather may still make the shoulder ache - use a hot pack!). At 1 year post-op you will have achieved the maximum functional recovery, with discomfort, range of movement and strength continuing to improve during this time.

◆ As with any joint replacement, it is unlikely that after a TSR you will have completely normal shoulder function. Expect some loss of range of movement compared to a normal shoulder. Some patients find it uncomfortable to sleep on that shoulder, and not all sports and leisure activities will be possible (or may be somewhat restricted).

Chapter 5

Choosing Your Surgeon

It is estimated that over 30,000 orthopaedic surgeons now operate in the US alone (there were 27,773 surgeons on record by the American Academy of Orthopaedic surgeons in 2012). So how do you even begin to choose an orthopaedic surgeon for your particular shoulder surgery?

After all, you should choose your orthopaedic surgeon as carefully as you choose your spouse! By working through the points in this chapter, you will be able to narrow your choice to one or two surgeons.

In your final choice, you must develop a strong working relationship with your surgeon and be confident of his/her abilities. Anxiety, distress, and lack of confidence in the procedure have all been shown to affect the successful outcome of elective orthopaedic surgery. Now is the time to start your progress to a highly successful outcome by choosing the orthopaedic surgeon who is right for *you*.

Referrals

◆ Your referring general practitioner or primary health physician can recommend local orthopaedic surgeons who have expertise in shoulder surgery, particularly your condition and procedure.

◆ Physical therapists with special expertise in rehabilitating shoulders post operatively will have an intimate knowledge of which shoulder orthopaedic surgeons have training and experience in your surgical procedure.

◆ Other health professionals with shoulder experience may also be able to recommend surgeons.

◆ Friends and relatives are often happy to recommend a surgeon they have had experience with, but be aware that well-meaning advice can lead you astray. If a particular surgeon is recommended, make sure the friend or relative has had the same or similar surgery. You need to compare oranges with oranges, not oranges with apples!

Online Research

Your surgeon's website & other websites (hospitals, professional associations) can provide a wealth of useful information:

◆ Where, when and how your surgeon was educated to achieve his qualifications as a surgeon.

◆ How is he qualified to be a surgeon? In the US, is he "Board Certified"? In other countries, is he a member of the Orthopaedic Surgeon's professional body?

◆ Experience—does your surgeon regularly

perform the type of shoulder surgery that you need?

◆ Does your surgeon have experience and training in the latest technology and techniques for this type of surgery?

◆ Gender—it is important to feel comfortable with the surgeon's gender as you will need to openly discuss personal information.

Hospital(s)

Which hospitals your surgeon operates at can be a deciding factor in your choice of surgeon.

◆ The convenience of a local hospital may be important to you.

◆ Also consider the reputation of the hospital, and ancillary facilities and services offered, such as physical therapy.

◆ Some hospitals offer residential post-operative rehabilitation, which can be important if you have no at-home support from family or friends.

◆ Call the hospital directly to enquire about costs of the procedure and all ancillary costs.

Fees vs Insurance Coverage

Contact your health insurer before approaching an orthopaedic surgeon, as there will most likely be out-of-pocket expenses. The choice of surgeon (and hospital) may minimise these expenses, but still consider the surgeon's qualifications, experience, and hospital reputation before finalising your choice.

The Initial Consultation

Be Prepared

This is the stage of the process that will determine the quality of relationship you build with the orthopaedic surgeon. Building this relationship will be easier if you go to this initial consultation well-prepared. By that I mean do your research (read this book!) and have some understanding of your condition. Go armed with a list of questions for the orthopaedic surgeon (see the chapter What You Need to Know from Your Orthopaedic Surgeon).

◆ It might also find it helpful to write out the course of the history of your shoulder problem in a simple bullet list. ◆ Keep these points concise and pertinent to your shoulder problem:

◆ List the aggravating factors and the level of pain.

◆ List the crucial points of the history of the shoulder in chronological order.

◆ List the treatments that you have had for the shoulder, their dates and effectiveness.

Arriving at this initial consultation well-prepared allows more time for answers to your list of questions.

Surgeon's Communication Style

During this initial consultation, the surgeon's communication skills and style will become apparent. If you find that you are comfortable with the style, and communication between you comes easily, then you have the solid basis of a working relationship. However, you are not looking for a new friend, but a competent professional who can communicate clearly with you.

Service level by other staff

Another factor that can determine whether the entire process (the lead up to your surgery, the surgery itself and your post-operative period) is smooth and stress free, is the level of service provided by the surgeon's ancillary staff, and their efficiency. Your experience with these staff members before and after this initial consultation should give you the clues you need to assess this.

Answers to your questions

It will be difficult after this initial consultation to remember all the answers that the surgeon has given you to your questions. I advise patients to take a friend or family member to listen to these answers and to take notes where appropriate. Having someone to confer with after the initial consultation also reduces the stress of the consultation itself, as you do not have to remember every single thing that the surgeon said.

Chapter 6

What Do You Need to Know from Your Surgeon?

C hoosing the right orthopaedic surgeon for your procedure is just the first step. Even more important is developing a good working relationship with the surgeon, and then learning everything you can from them about why this procedure is chosen, the process for this procedure, and the expected ultimate outcome.

Each and every time you visit your orthopaedic surgeon is an opportunity for you both to develop a working relationship and good communication.

More importantly these consultations, especially the first, are your opportunity to gather information and have all your questions answered. You must attend these consultations well-prepared.

The initial consultation will be far more productive if you have to hand all the information that the orthopaedic surgeon will need:

◆ The referral from your primary physician or general practitioner.

◆ A listing of your previous medical history, especially any operations. Don't rely on the referral from your medical practitioner to

BRUCE PAULIK

have listed everything. On the day, you will forget important facts without this list.

◆ Copies of any imaging reports or pathology reports that you have available.

◆ A complete list of all current prescription and over-the-counter medications.

◆ A brief summary of your current symptoms and limitations on using the shoulder.

Now your initial consultation will flow smoothly and efficiently, leaving enough time for all your questions.

My advice to every patient is to take a friend or relative with you for your initial consultation with the orthopaedic surgeon. You will not remember everything that is said, so your friend or relative will sit with you and compare notes later.

So what do you need to know from your orthopaedic surgeon and what are the questions to ask to gather this information?

◆ What are my alternatives to surgery? Have I exhausted all nonsurgical or minimally invasive treatment options? Are there any treatment options that we should try first, such as injections or physical therapy?

◆ Given my current physical and medical condition, am I a suitable candidate for surgery? If not what treatment options do I have?

◆ What surgical procedure is being recommended, and what are the options for other procedures?

◆ How is this procedure done and what sort of anaesthesia will I need?

◆ How soon before I can drive after surgery?

◆ What is the recovery period, and how soon will I be able to return to work and sport?

◆ What post-operative rehabilitation program will be needed for this procedure?

◆ Would I benefit from a pre-operative rehab program? (see the chapter "Prehab before Rehab")

◆ What is the success rate for this procedure, and what will the ultimate outcome be in terms of pain and function? Will I be able to return to all sports, work and leisure activities eventually?

◆ What are the risks and possible complications of this procedure?

◆ Is there printed information available describing the procedure and the postoperative recovery?

◆ What is your experience with this operation?

I can't over-emphasise the importance of the information that you get from your orthopaedic surgeon at this initial consultation and any later consultations. What this book provides is an overview of the process and highlights the important issues—it sets you in the right direction. What the surgeon can provide are the specifics of your operation, and his guidance and advice on the timing of your rehabilitation program.

Each patient's procedure is specific to them, and each surgeon has a preferred timeline for the progress of your rehabilitation based on the specifics of the procedure. So the information you get from the surgeon both **before** the operation and **after** the operation is a vital component of your rehabilitation process. You can see that developing good communication with the surgeon is vital.

Chapter 7

Prehab before Rehab

S o you have committed to that shoulder surgery. You have all the information you need from the surgeon and a firm date for the surgery. By now you understand the post-operative rehabilitation process.

But you have probably been favouring that painful shoulder for quite some time now and pain has limited your activity. That means reduced range of motion, weak and tight muscles, poorer general fitness and perhaps even some weight gain. Should you do anything between now and the surgery? Absolutely!

A physiotherapist can design a prehabilitation exercise program specific to the needs of *your* shoulder, starting 2 to 6 weeks before your surgery, to achieve:

Improved range of motion of the shoulder

Your range of shoulder movement can be restricted by several factors, such as:

♦ pain,

♦ tightness of the glenohumeral joint capsule, and

◆ tightness of any combination of muscles around the shoulder.

You can relieve the joint capsule tightness and muscular tightness with the right combination of exercises. This will lead to a marked improvement in your active range of movement, with less pain caused by these movements.

Shoulder problems respond well to "active/assisted" exercises suitable for your shoulder. An example of active/assisted exercises is gripping the fingers of both hands together and using the stronger arm to take the weaker/painful arm into forward elevation (either sitting, standing or lying). You can use a rope and pulley system for a similar effect.

It's also possible that some gentle manual therapy techniques by the physical therapist will help achieve these goals.

Going into your shoulder surgery with better range of movement and less pain will certainly affect the speed of your recovery from surgery. This is why patients are now being sent for a prehabilitation program before many types of orthopaedic surgery.

Improved strength of the rotator cuff muscles.

Pain and swelling from shoulder inflammation produce reflex inhibition and weakening of the muscles controlling the shoulder joint, in particular the rotator cuff muscles.

Before surgery, neuromuscular control needs to be restored to improve muscle function post-operatively. To put it simply: you need to wake up these muscles! The better the control you have of these muscles, and the stronger they are, the better the post-operative recovery process.

Prehabilitation strengthening exercises for the rotator cuff muscles could start with isometric contractions (gentle sustained holds against light resistance with no movement). These can then progress to isotonic exercises (exercises against light resistance with movement). Your physical therapist can show you the correct exercises to do that will not aggravate your shoulder condition.

Improve strength and activation of the scapular stabilising muscles.

As a result of shoulder pain and stiffness over a lengthy period, the body will have most likely developed abnormal movement patterns in an attempt to take the load off the painful shoulder. Weak, stiff or unstable shoulders will often develop a compensatory pattern of overusing the upper trapezius muscle, with the other lower stabilising muscles of the scapula becoming weaker.

This muscle imbalance contributes to increasing shoulder pain and stress on the neck and upper back, with pain and stiffness experienced in these areas. Experiencing these symptoms secondary to a painful shoulder is very common where symptoms have been ongoing for months or years.

A prehabilitation exercise program to relax the upper trapezius and engage the other scapula stabilising muscles will set you up for a much easier postoperative rehabilitation program.

Understand and learn the early post-operative routine and exercises.

During your prehabilitation program is the perfect time to learn how to do your early post-operative exercises. Immediately after the surgery when you have shoulder pain is not the best time to be learning new exercises.

The exercises you perform in the first 2 to 4 weeks will aim at maintaining shoulder range of movement and the scapular stability, with the limitations imposed by the surgeon. Learning the correct technique for these exercises and practising them during the prehabilitation program will give you immeasurable confidence in the immediate post-operative period.

Learn how to protect the shoulder post-operatively and the correct way to apply and use the sling.

In the prehabilitation program, your physical therapist will instruct you on how to put on and wear the type of sling that you will require post-operatively. It is important that you apply and remove this sling in the correct manner so you don't overstress the operative site.

With certain types of surgery, such as rotator cuff repairs, you will need to learn how to move the shoulder with the help of the other arm or gravity, placing no stress on the repaired tendons. Applying your sling correctly and moving the arm and shoulder correctly can go a long way to making your post-operative period much less painful.

Each surgeon will have their own protocol for the post-operative period, which will place certain limitations on allowed movements and activities. During the prehabilitation program the physical therapist will go through the surgeon's post-operative protocol so you are clear about what the limitations on shoulder movement and exercise are for your procedure.

Become mentally prepared for the post-operative period.

Often patients are nervous about their shoulder surgery, and may have forgotten to ask the surgeon all the questions that they would like answered, or may have thought of new questions.

The Prehab program allows the therapist to:

◆ explain the procedure in some detail,

◆ answer the forgotten questions,

◆ go over preparations immediately prior to the surgery, and

◆ explain the post-operative rehabilitation process in complete detail.

This process can allay your nervousness and build a positive mental attitude to your recovery from surgery. This is often the most important benefit you will gain from the Prehab program.

Chapter 8

Prepare for Surgery

You have signed up for the shoulder surgery, a date has been set and you have started your prehabilitation program. Everything is under control. But is it?

The surgeon will have advised you about the post-operative process and timing. You will be "out of action" for a time, depending on the type of surgery. Now is the time to think through the post-op period and put in place your plans to cope with just one shoulder working normally.

Post-op Assistance

You will need help during the post-op period for anything from a few days to a few weeks, depending on the type of surgery and how long you will need to wear your sling. If you normally live alone, organise a friend or family member to stay with you for 1 to 7 days, until you feel comfortable coping with the normal activities of daily living with one arm in the sling. The first 24 hours is particularly vital to have help to get settled. Otherwise talk through this issue of personal assistance with members of your normal household.

You will require this personal assistance from—or in fact total dependence on—this friend or family member for a wide range of daily tasks such as showering, dressing and food preparation. Even simple tasks such as eating, moving from sitting to standing, toileting can be problematic in the first few post-operative days.

Prepare Your Home

In the days leading up to your surgery it is beneficial to imagine how you will cope with every single activity of daily living with one arm out of action. This is especially applicable where you will be unable to place any strain whatsoever on the shoulder e.g. after rotator cuff repair or total shoulder replacement.

The best way to approach this is to put your arm in a temporary sling and spend some hours at home going through all of your daily activities. You will soon see where the difficulties lie and where you will need help from your personal assistant (family member or friend), or where you will need to modify the activity or purchase items to make these activities easier.

Some examples of simple items that you can purchase or hire:

◆ Shower chair—you will be able to sit and shower without fear of falling or over-stressing your operated shoulder. In the post-operative period you will feel weak and perhaps even dizzy. A shower chair will make the entire process more comfortable and safer.

◆ Detachable showerhead—as you must keep your incision dry for a period post-operatively, a detachable showerhead makes this easily achievable especially if you use a waterproof dressing (please note that these dressings are not always 100% waterproof!).

◆ Waterproof dressings and surgical tape.

◆ Toiletries easy to use one-handed. Keep toiletries in the shower and on the bathroom bench within easy reach.

◆ Slip resistant mats where necessary such as in the shower or bathtub, or on the bathroom floor.

◆ Pillows—having extra pillows and cushions will be useful for propping your arm up when you're sitting on the couch or lying in bed.

◆ Reclining pillows—if you have trouble getting comfortable with your shoulder at night post operatively you may find it's best to semi recline with the purpose made pillows or foam blocks. For the best quality sleep, sleep experts recommend lying back at an angle of at most 40°. You may prefer to sleep in a reclining armchair with the operated arm supported by pillows.

◆ Frozen meal packs—naturally we all prefer to eat food cooked from fresh ingredients for each meal. At a time like this you will be thankful to have some frozen meal packs available for those moments when you are just not up to cooking. You can also make some of your favourite soups and meals and freeze them in advance. You might also consider a meals home delivery service.

◆ Medicine supply box—you can have your medications set out in the right order at the right time of the day so that you won't be forgetting to take your meds or taking more than you should. Your pharmacist can also organise this for you in a weekly "blister pack".

◆ Additions to your wardrobe—you need to have front opening shirts and jackets, preferably slightly overlarge for ease of use with an arm that you're restricted from moving normally.

Hazard-proof Your Home

In the post-op period it's absolutely vital that you don't stumble and fall at home. Landing on the arm or shoulder could seriously disrupt the surgeon's work. Even a stumble without falling can cause you to jerk your shoulder suddenly, leading to a marked increase in pain and stiffness, even without damaging the surgical site.

Patients are reminded constantly of the need to protect their shoulder post-operatively from certain active movements. But in my experience of several decades of rehabilitating patients' shoulders, the most common reason for damaging the shoulder post-operatively is falling over. Eliminating all trip hazards before surgery is therefore time very well spent.

Examine your home carefully for trip hazards:

◆ One of the worst trip hazards in most homes are rugs on the floor—it's so easy to catch a toe on the edge of a rug, especially when you're not at your most agile self post-operatively.

◆ Cables that extend across walkways should be re-routed to a safer place.

◆ The bathroom is certainly a high hazard dangerous area—the floor is often tiled, and when combined with water is an accident waiting to happen. Look at your process in the bathroom and practice with one arm in a sling. You'll soon notice how easy it would be to slip over. Do you need and rails installed in a couple of key spots? Do you need nonslip mats on the shower or bathtub floor?

◆ Check all pathways around your house and have any raised edges repaired.

◆ If you have steps at your home, are the handrails secure and not loose. If you have steps without a handrail, do you need to have a hand rail installed?

◆ Dimly lit or unlit areas around your home can increase the risk of falls night. Consider setting up lamps or nightlights to cover these areas. Avoid walking in dark areas around your house at night, especially in the immediate post-operative period when your balance may be affected.

◆ Keep any glasses or contact lenses within easy reach—you do not want to be fumbling around for them, and you especially don't want to be walking around the house with poor vision. For convenience, consider purchasing an extra pair of glasses.

◆ In the kitchen set up your groceries, crockery and cooking utensils within easy reach. You want to avoid either bending down low or even worse stepping up onto a footstool to reach high items.

◆ Socks and slippers without tread don't provide adequate traction on slippery surfaces and should be avoided.

Personal Preparation

And there is still more you can do to be prepared!

◆ Pay all bills—both those currently owing and for the next month if possible. This way you won't be handling payments in the immediate post-op period when you won't be at your sharpest mentally!

◆ Give someone written authority to pick up medications from your pharmacy—you may need to speak to your pharmacy to arrange this.

◆ Write out a list of important telephone numbers—both for yourself and anyone assisting you. This should include your orthopaedic surgeon, general physician, pharmacy and family members.

◆ Bring all household chores such as washing and cleaning up to date—you are not going to be fit enough to do any strenuous activity, and you will be less likely to overstress your shoulder.

◆ As you will be "taking it easy" for a period, make sure that you have organised your entertainment—books, TV series, films. You need to set up a comfortable supportive armchair, footrest and side table (on your good side) with all these entertainment items within reach. Keep a good supply of pillows to support your arm within reach.

◆ For the first week or two you may find it more comfortable sleeping in a reclining armchair at night with your arm supported by pillows. Apparently to get good quality sleep you should recline at no more than 40° off horizontal, that is the closer to horizontal the better!

Transport

As you will not be allowed to drive post-operatively for a period, depending on your type of surgery, consider the following situations.

◆ You will need to be driven home after the

surgery—in fact you cannot leave the hospital unescorted. You need to have someone stay with you for at least 24 hours after the surgery—especially applicable for day surgery patients who go home the day of the procedure.

◆ Your surgeon will give you guidelines about your return to driving yourself, but this can be up to 2 months. You must not drive until given the go ahead by your surgeon or physiotherapist. You risk the integrity of the shoulder procedure if you drive too early, and you can be a risk to yourself and others if you are not physically ready.

◆ You will need to organise transport for appointments eg for post-op physiotherapy and surgeon consultations.

Prepare Your Work

It is important in the immediate post-op period that you can devote your energies to recovery. If you are needed to have repeated input to your work by phone or email, then you are not focusing on recovery!

◆ If you run your own business, delegate your responsibilities to others—business partners, employees. Reschedule meetings, trips, conferences to free up the post-op period. Put in the extra work *before* the surgery, so that you are not needed for a period *after* the surgery!

◆ As an employee, sit down with your manager to delegate important work while you are away, and organise a *sensible* return to work schedule based on your surgeon's advice. Allow more time than you think you might need—you will be surprised how long it takes to feel up to returning to work.

Chapter 9

The Day Arrives!

Finally! The big day is here—there are some things that you have been aware of over the past few days, and you will have specific instructions for today:

Food, Drink & Medication

◆ You have stopped taking all medications that cause blood thinning (unless otherwise advised by your surgeon) and for the past week you have stopped taking all herbal remedies, aspirin and anti-inflammatory medications.

◆ Since midnight last night you have consumed no food or liquids, including mints and chewing gum. It's probably not advisable to smoke or consume alcohol in the 24 hours before surgery.

◆ You will have been advised which medications are permissible to take this morning—take them with just a small sip of water.

◆ If you are experiencing any noticeable change in your health today, such as coughing and elevated temperature, notify your doctor immediately.

Hygiene and Dress

- ◆ It's permissible to brush your teeth prior to surgery but don't swallow any liquid.

- ◆ Jewellery and body piercings should not be worn to surgery.

- ◆ Don't take valuables or electronics to hospital with you, unless you have someone to leave them with.

- ◆ If you wear glasses, dentures bring a container to put them in when you remove them.

- ◆ Wear comfortable loose clothing and make sure that you have a front opening fairly loose button-up shirt to wear after surgery. Wear flat sold slip-on shoes that don't require lacing up.

- ◆ If you have been given the sling to wear after the surgery, remember to bring with you.

- ◆ Think about your comfort in the vehicle on the way home—supportive pillows and a blanket can help.

- ◆ And just a reminder—is the person who is providing transport there and back able to stay with you for the first 24 hours when you get home?

What Happens at the Hospital?

Although the details will vary depending on your surgical procedure and the hospital, the basic steps will be:

- ◆ When you present to reception, any final paperwork will be completed.

- ◆ You will be shown to pre-op waiting area and asked to change into a surgical gown. Your clothes and belongings will be secured.

- ◆ The nursing staff will take certain measurements such as height, weight, temperature, pulse and blood pressure. If you have diabetes, they will do a blood glucose test.

- ◆ The anaesthesia provider may visit you for a final check.

- ◆ A healthcare practitioner will mark the shoulder to be operated on.

- ◆ You will be commenced on your anaesthesia—either regional or general, or both.

Immediately Following Surgery

It's not uncommon for many people to go home on the day of their surgery. This will depend on the type of surgery—the surgeon will allow you to go home as soon as it is safe for you.

Here's what to expect from the process:

◆ Immediately after the surgery, the healthcare staff will take you to a recovery area and monitor you until your anaesthesia wears off. Your family and friends are often allowed to visit once you're awake. At this point you're either deemed well enough to go home, or moved to your inpatient room if you're staying overnight.

◆ You will be given medication to provide pain control. You should expect there to be some pain, but the medication should keep this pain within tolerable limits. They may also give you a cold pack for the shoulder to help control pain and post-operative swelling. (See the chapter Managing Pain.)

◆ In most cases, they will give you a sling to wear in the post-operative period (see the chapter Living with a Sling). The type of sling and how long you will be required to wear it will depend on your surgery. Before you leave the hospital, you must understand the correct way to put the sling on and off and how to adjust it.

◆ Be aware that the combination of your anaesthesia, food and car motion can cause nausea and vomiting. If you're going home on the day of your surgery, it's probably best to wait until you arrive home before eating. Begin with a light meal and avoid greasy food.

Chapter 10

Living with a Sling

After shoulder surgery, it is most likely that you will need to wear a sling over your clothes for 2 to 6 weeks. For simple surgery like arthroscopic acromioplasty, the sling will be used to rest the shoulder for 1 to 2 weeks to allow post-operative soreness to settle. In this case, you will be encouraged to remove the sling and move the arm gently during this period.

On the other hand, if you've had a procedure that requires extensive healing post-operatively, it becomes crucial that you keep the arm supported in

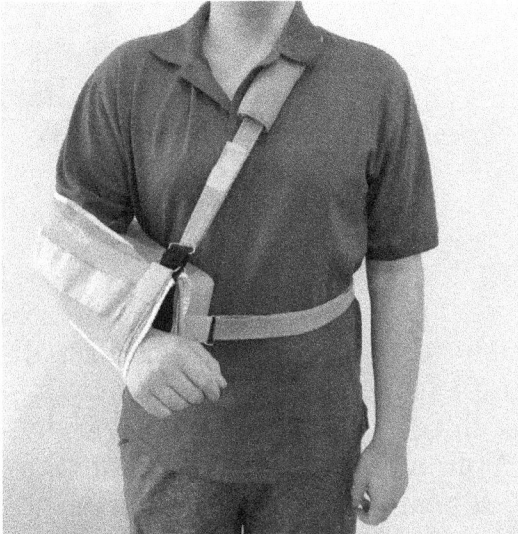

the sling for the period advised by the orthopaedic surgeon. For instance, after rotator cuff repair it's likely that you'll wear the sling for 4 to 6 weeks.

The type of sling that you wear will vary—if you have had a rotator cuff repair, it is most likely that you will wear an *abduction sling* (as above). This has a cushion underneath the arm to hold it away from the body. The purpose of this abduction sling is to relieve the tension on the repaired rotator cuff tendons for up to 6 weeks to allow initial healing to take place.

For other types of surgery, a *simple broad arm sling* is used—this allows the arm to rest against the body:

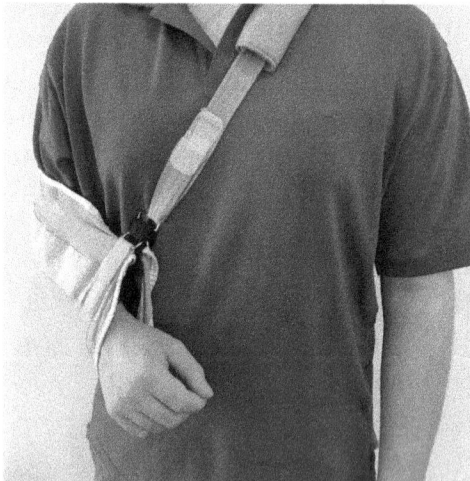

If you have been advised to wear your sling continuously (e.g. after rotator cuff repair or total shoulder replacement) then be certain to support the arm in the sling position when getting dressed and washing. Your sling should stay on at all times, day and night, to maintain the protection of the repaired tissues in the shoulder.

However, it is essential that you remove or loosen the sling 3 to 4 times daily to exercise the elbow, wrist and hand. This will maintain the flexibility of these joints. Your surgeon or physiotherapist will have given you a protocol to follow, outlining the exercises to do. Alternatively, just do the simple exercises listed here.

Simple exercises while wearing a sling

Practise these exercises at least 3 times per day with 10 repetitions of each exercise, depending on shoulder pain.

◆ Stretch your fingers open and then close your fist, progressing to squeezing a soft ball. Also stretch the thumb across your hand and out to the side.

◆ Bend your wrist back and forwards. Twist your forearm/hand down and then up.

◆ Lying on your back with the elbow supported on a pillow bent double, undo the forearm straps on the sling - bend then fully straighten your elbow. Please note that an elbow can get very stiff while bent to right angles in your sling, so this movement is important. You don't want elbow stiffness to be a major problem during your shoulder rehabilitation period!

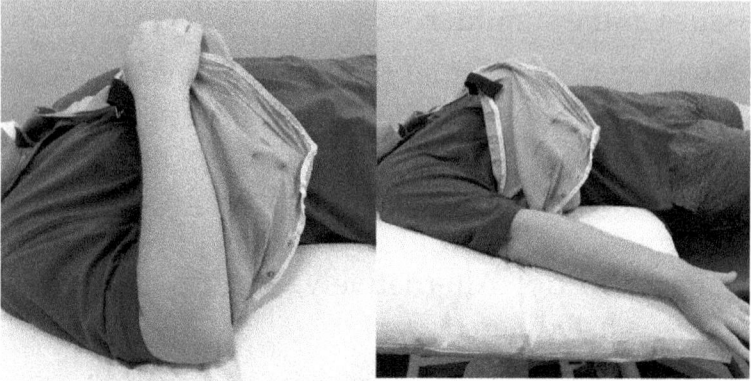

◆ Shoulder retractions - sit with your arms supported on your lap (sling on). Pull your shoulder blades back together and down, hold 5 seconds. Don't pull back hard enough to cause shoulder pain.

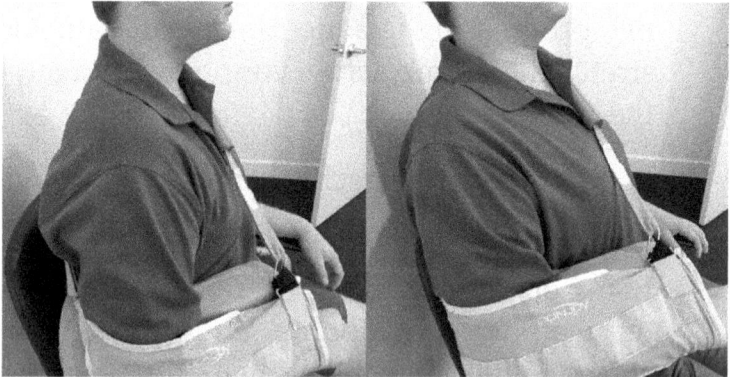

If you're wearing a sling continuously to protect the shoulder you will need some help at first with washing and dressing. It's best to wear loose tops that button down the front, and loose pants or skirt that are easy to step into. Women may find bra straps uncomfortable - strapless or front fastening may be preferable.

Slip-on shoes are essential—no need to be reaching down to try to lace up shoes with one hand! I have lost count of the hundreds of times over my years of rehabilitating shoulders that I have needed to help patients on with their shoes and lace them up for them. To avoid falls, make sure that your slip-on shoes are safe and not slippery.

Putting your sling on

With assistance:

If you are required to wear your sling at all times to protect the healing tissues (e.g. after rotator cuff repair or total shoulder replacement), you may find it easier in the first 2 weeks to put the sling on with assistance.

Support the operated arm with your opposite hand with the elbow bent. Your assistant will slide the sling on from behind the elbow until your elbow is completely into the sling.

If you are wearing an abduction sling, the arm should be supported away from the body during this manoeuvre in the position it will adopt once in the sling. You may prefer to sit with the arm supported on a pillow. Then follow the instruction as below, but with assistance.

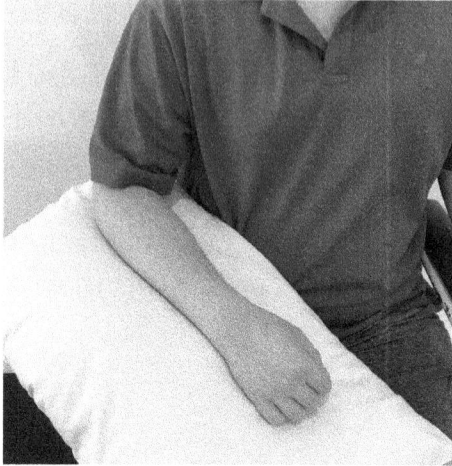

Without assistance:

Now it is definitely better to be seated, with the elbow bent to 90 degrees and the forearm supported on a pillow

Slide the sling on from behind the elbow with the opposite hand - do not actively support the weight of the operated arm with its own muscles. Fasten the strap across your forearm.

With your opposite hand reach the shoulder strap where it is attached to the elbow part of the sling, and take it behind your neck and across the opposite shoulder. Attach the Velcro fastener at the front, tight enough so that the forearm is supported horizontal.

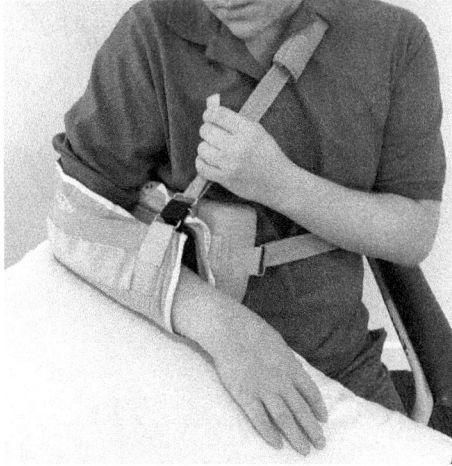

Now take the waist belt around your back and attach to the front of the sling - just tight enough to support the sling comfortably against your body.

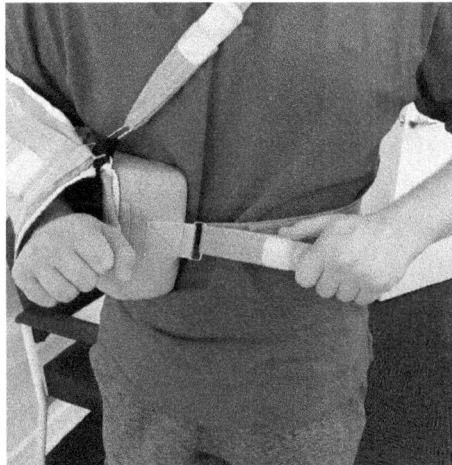

The end result should be comfortable, supported but not tight. Do *not* adjust the sling to pull your arm hard across the front of your body.

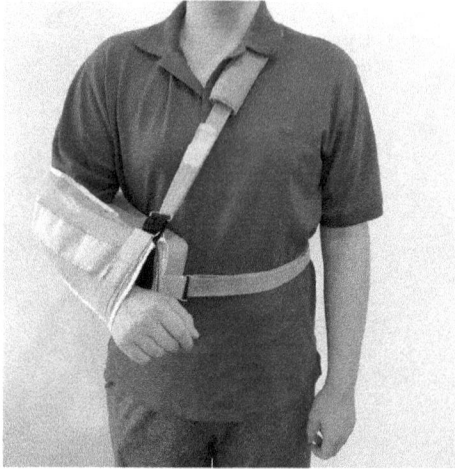

Taking your sling off

Sit with your arm supported on a pillow.

Remove the waist and neck straps with the opposite hand, being careful not to move or lift the operated arm. Using your opposite hand, slide the sling out from under the elbow.

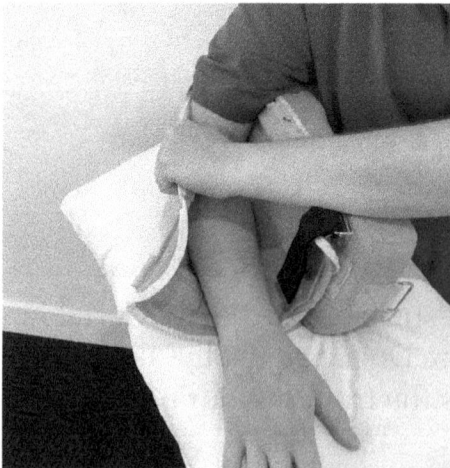

Chapter 11

Managing Pain after Surgery

L et's be realistic right from the start. You will experience pain post-operatively, and this pain will vary considerably depending on the type of surgery you have had, and your individual response to the surgery.

Even within the same individual, pain from a particular procedure can vary from one time to another. This postoperative pain can last for a variable period - days through to months. The amount of pain, swelling, bruising and inflammation will vary enormously. So I want to talk to you in this chapter about managing the pain, swelling and inflammation post-operatively.

It's important to understand that you will be *managing* the pain, and that the medication you take will *not* give you complete relief of your pain. But in this chapter I have described other methods to supplement the pain medication.

There may be those of you who want to "tough it out" because you believe you have a high pain tolerance. Very few of us have the high pain tolerance we think we have. This is not the right approach. If you don't keep the pain under control and at manageable levels, then any or all of the following will occur:

- ◆ You will be unable to carry out your post-op exercises effectively.

- ◆ Muscles around the shoulder girdle, neck and upper back will become overactive and tight, causing pain in these areas.

- ◆ The shoulder will be stiffer than expected, and return to good range of movement will be delayed.

- ◆ During your rehabilitation process, the return of muscle strength around the shoulder will be delayed.

As part of your anaesthesia for the surgery, you may have had a nerve block. This is an anaesthetic injection into the major nerves leaving the neck. This leaves the shoulder and arm numb and pain-free for up to 12 hours after the surgery. When this wears off the shoulder pain can kick in quickly, and you will need effective strong painkillers. In hospital, you will need to inform nursing staff as soon as this pain starts.

The first 2 to 4 weeks after surgery will be the critical period for good pain management. It's during this period that you will experience the most pain and will need a consistent approach to your medication. The correct approach is to take the simple painkillers (see below) regularly at the prescribed daily dose, and then top up with stronger opioid type painkillers as needed (see below).

Types of Pain-killing Medication after Surgery

Please note that all comments below about medication are general in nature, and you will need to follow your surgeon's advice concerning postoperative medication.

Simple Pain-killers (taken regularly):

◆ **Paracetamol** (acetaminophen; trade names: Panadol, Tylenol, others).
Paracetamol is a simple and effective painkiller. It is very safe if you stay within the recommended maximum daily dosage, with virtually no side effects. It is usually taken every 4 to 6 hours. It works best if taken at regular intervals - don't just wait until the pain is unbearable and then expect the Paracetamol to bring the pain under control. An effective regime is two 500mg tablets after each meal and then two before bed.

◆ **Non- Steroidal Anti-inflammatory Medications** ("NSAIDs"; trade names: Nurofen, Voltaren, Celebrex, Mobic, Feldene, Brufen, many others).
NSAIDs, apart from an anti-inflammatory effect (including reduced swelling and soreness), are effective in pain relief. They have been shown to be even more effective in postoperative pain relief when combined with Paracetamol. They may also be used in conjunction with opioids for more severe pain..
As NSAIDs can cause indigestion or reflux,

they should always be taken with food. Each type of NSAID will have a different dose and frequency, and should be taken as prescribed. They are generally very safe for periods up to 30 days, but should only be taken on advice from your surgeon or general physician post-operatively.

Opioid Painkillers (taken as needed):

For moderate to severe postoperative pain, where the regular use of Paracetamol and NSAID's is not sufficient, then you may be prescribed one of the various narcotic analgesics to supplement your usual daily medications. These are for short term use to reduce the most severe postoperation pain. As they can be addictive, you stop taking them as soon as the pain settles enough for the Paracetamol and NSAID's to be enough.

Common postoperative opioids:

◆ **Paracetamol with codeine** (eg Panadeine and Panadeine Forte). The same limits apply as for Paracetamol alone so that you don't go over the daily maximum for Paracetamol. Codeine is unfortunately likely to cause constipation - keep up your fluids and dietary fibre to help minimize this.

◆ **Tramadol** (eg Tramal, Ultram) is a synthetic opioid commonly prescribed post-operatively in combination with Paracetamol or NSAID's. Take only as directed. Do not start taking other medication without checking with your physician. It may be supplied as a slow release version for longer acting affect.

◆ **Oxycodone** (eg Endone, OxyContin) is a very strong painkiller used for severe pain. It is available in immediate release and slow release forms.

◆ **Analgesic patches** (eg Norspan, Fentanyl) can be used to give a steady supply of the relevant painkiller over a five-day period after they are applied. Only one should be applied at any one time. It may take up to twelve hours for the maximum effect of the patch, and as many hours for the drug to wear off if it is removed.

◆ **Drugs supplied by intravenous drip in hospital** (eg Morphine, Pethidine, Fentanyl). These are usually only required in the first 24 hours after surgery. The medication may be supplied by Patent Controlled Analgesia - a computerised pump supplies the medication to an intravenous drip up to a predetermined maximum. The patient decides when they need more medication by pressing a button. You cannot take too much as the maximum has been set by the doctor. You will be under observation in hospital, and the nursing staff will need to check your blood pressure regularly—and wake you in the process!

◆ **Pregabalin** (eg Lyrica) is commonly used to treat neuropathic (nerve) pain

Alternative Methods to Help Manage Postoperative Pain

Cryotherapy

Cryotherapy is the use of cold therapy (as in ice packs) to assist in pain management and control of inflammation and swelling. Studies have shown that cryotherapy for shoulders in the postoperative period helps control pain, decreases swelling and muscle spasm, and suppresses inflammation. Patients report less pain and better sleep in the immediate postoperative period (0 to 3 days). With continued use over the next 10 days patients report other benefits such as less swelling, easier movement and less pain during rehabilitation exercises.

Simple readily available cold or ice packs are the most economic, but you can also purchase commercial cryotherapy products especially shaped to the shoulder (eg Cryocuff, Game Ready).

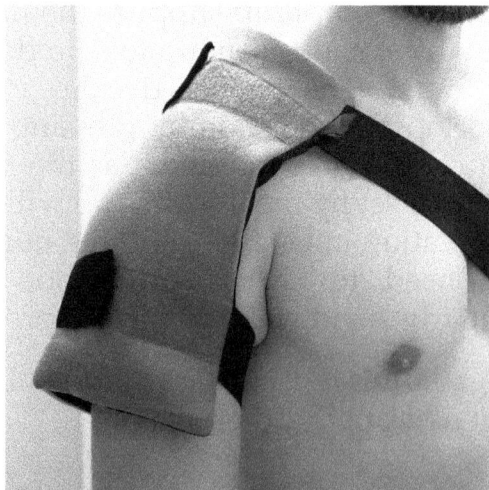

How to use cryotherapy:

Apply an ice pack for 20 minutes every two hours while awake during days 0 to 3. Continue over days 2 to 14 for up to 20 minutes every hour as needed. Never apply the icepack directly to the skin as it can cause skin damage (a "cold burn"), but rather have a layer of cloth between the icepack and the skin. Also don't apply the icepack to an area where the skin is numb.

Cryotherapy is also useful during rehabilitation—it can be used over the shoulder after an exercise session to reduce post exercise discomfort and swelling.

Heat

Local heat ("thermotherapy") should never be used in the early postoperative period (the first 2 to 3 weeks) as it can cause increased bleeding and swelling.

Later, as you progress through the rehabilitation period, using local heat by applying a hot pack over the shoulder can improve circulation, relax tight muscles and relieve pain. Used before exercise, the heat allows more effective stretching and exercising, resulting in a faster return of your range of motion.

TENS

Transcutaneous Electrical Nerve Stimulation (TENS) is a method of pain relief in which a small battery operated electrical device provides a low-level electrical stimulation to the skin in the area of pain via small electrodes attached to the skin. This electrical stimulation causes a warm tingling sensation which passes into your nervous system. It is thought to relieve pain by competing with the pain signals in the spinal cord for transmission through to the brain (the "Gate Theory" of pain modulation). This causes reduction in the pain and relaxation of muscle spasm.

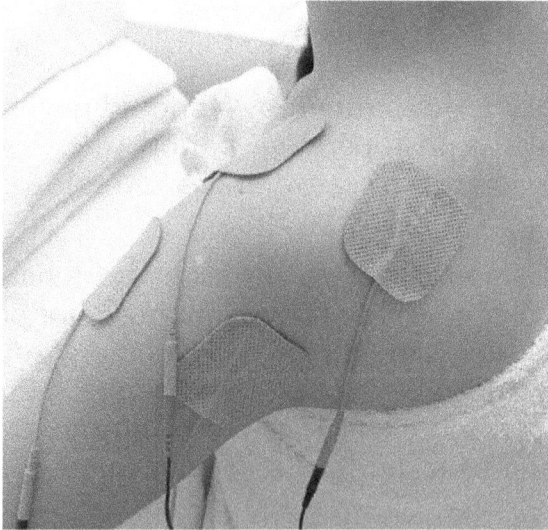

TENS is applied in periods of between 5 and 30 minutes to help manage peak periods of pain. Do not use TENS if you have an implanted medical device (eg cardiac pacemaker).

Gentle Passive Movement

Gentle early passive movement of the operated shoulder is a valuable and essential component of the healing and recovery process. In my experience patients report that the shoulder feels far more comfortable after gentle therapist-supported passive movement within pain-free limits. As each procedure has its own restrictions, please adhere strictly to your surgeon/physiotherapist's advice. You may be allowed to carry out early gentle "auto-assisted" passive movements where the operated arm is supported by the opposite arm.

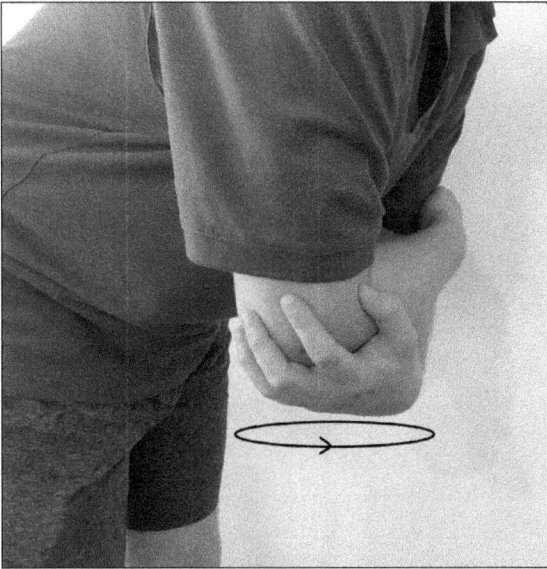

Gentle soft tissue massage

Your shoulder pain will cause increased muscle tension throughout the neck, upper back and shoulder girdle on the operated side. Muscles that are commonly tight post-operatively include trapezius, the rotator cuff muscles, latissimus dorsi, teres major, deltoids and the pectorals. This tightness in turn restricts your recovery and leads to a further increase in your pain.

Gentle massage to release this muscular tension will pay immediate dividends in the amount of pain you experience, and the ease of performing your rehabilitation exercises.

Your physiotherapist is best qualified to perform these gentle soft tissue release techniques in the early postoperative stages.

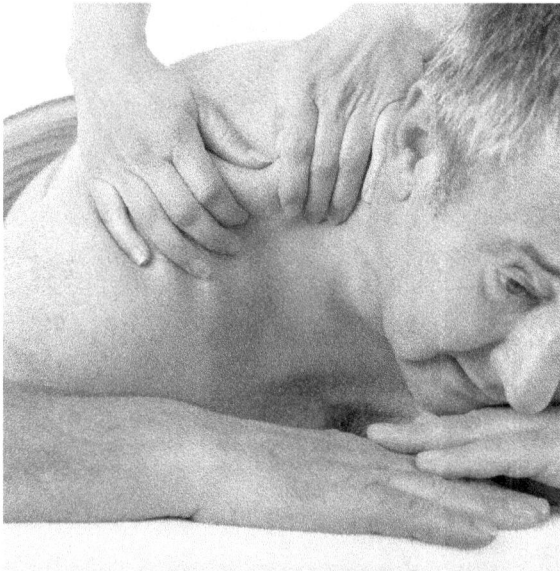

Acupuncture

Traditional Chinese acupuncture involves the insertion of very fine needles into specific acupuncture points, depending on the area being treated. It is thought to relieve pain by stimulating the release of endorphins, which are your body's natural pain-killing hormones.

Acupuncture has been shown to be effective in relieving musculoskeletal pain, especially when combined with analgesic medications.

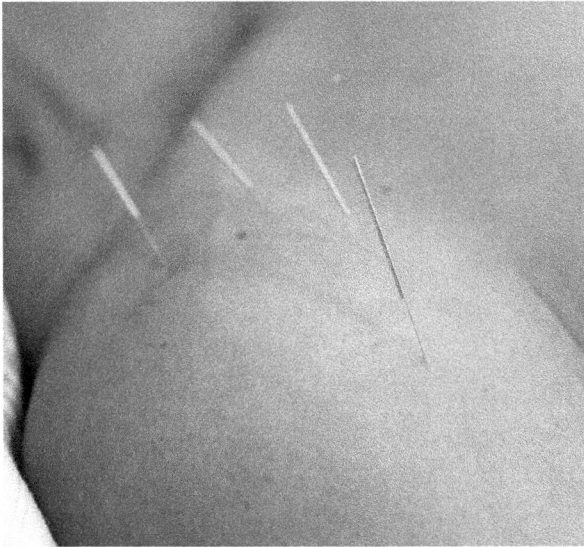

Meditation, hypnosis and relaxation techniques

These could all be classed as psychological methods of pain control. There is evidence to support the use of these techniques to supplement your postoperative medication. In an analysis of 18 studies of the use of medical hypnosis, guided imagery, or relaxation techniques, researchers showed improvement in both physical and emotional postsurgical recovery.

Chapter 12

Managing at Home

T his is where all the preparation you did before your surgery pays dividends. If you have followed my instructions in the chapter "Prepare for Surgery" then you should have some strategies in place for managing day-to-day activities using only one arm. This chapter will also cover most common daily activities with tips and strategies for coping.

Of course, how much you are allowed to do with your operated arm will depend on the surgical procedure. If at one end of the scale you have had an arthroscopic acromioplasty, you will wear a sling for 1 to 2 weeks and using the arm as much as pain allows. If on the other hand you have had a shoulder replacement or rotator cuff repair, you will wear a sling for 4 to 6 weeks and have instructions which severely limit the use of that arm. For the discussion about daily activities that follows, I will assume the most restricted permissible use of the operated arm.

Washing/showering

◆ For the first couple of weeks, you will be well advised to wash/shower seated as you may feel weak and unsteady at first. You can use a shower chair, or sit on a bath board that sits snugly across the bath.

◆ If you have had a rotator cuff repair and been advised to not allow the arm to sit against your side, you will wear an abduction sling. When you shower, you may need to use a small pillow wrapped in plastic under your elbow to hold your arm slightly away from your body.

◆ If you need to step into a bath while your arm is in a sling, be certain you have a handrail for your non-operated arm, and a non-slip bath mat. In my experience, the most common cause of damage to the operated shoulder is a fall.

Dressing/undressing

◆ *Dress your operated arm first and undress it last.* You may find it helpful to have an assistant in the first two or three weeks until your shoulder pain has settled and you become adept at managing the process. Remember that if you are in an abduction sling, you must keep your arm supported away from your side—no lower than the position in the sling.

◆ *Tops:* wear loose-fitting tops, preferably with buttons down the front. Small buttons and fastenings should be avoided. If the top does not button down the front, it will need to be very loose and preferably short sleeved.

◆ *Wearing a bra:* women may find it easier to use a front opening bra and/or a strapless bra. If using a normal bra, it may be best to do up the rear fastenings, then step into it and pull it up over the hips with the unaffected arm, slipping arms into the straps as it's pulled up. All fastening must be done only with the unaffected arm throughout the dressing and undressing process.

◆ *Undressing:* sit with the arm supported on a pillow, then remove the sling (see the chapter "Living with a Sling"). Undo the front buttons and slip your sleeve off the unaffected arm. This arm is now free to slide the sleeve off the operated arm. Wear comfortable loose-fitting pants, eg track pants that will slide down easily once released at the waist. Keep that operated arm well supported throughout the process!

◆ *Dressing:* again sit with the arm supported on a pillow. Using the unaffected arm (and an assistant if available) slide the sleeve up the operated arm and across the shoulder, continuing the motion to slide the unaffected arm into its sleeve. Put on the sling (see the chapter "Living with a Sling"). Slip your feet into your pants or skirt, pulling them up as far as possible while seated. Stand and then complete pulling up the pants. Slip into your slip-on shoes. All done!

Kitchen/meals

◆ *Meal preparation:* for the first few weeks use pre-prepared meals (perhaps you were busy cooking and freezing before your surgery?) or meals that require minimal preparation. This is when meal delivery services are very convenient. It is important that you eat well and healthily for best healing of your shoulder. For the first 4 to 6 weeks you must use your unoperated arm only for all kitchen and meal activities. There is a range of helpful kitchen items available to help with single-handed chores eg single-handed jar openers. Browse kitchen supply shops for these.

◆ *Meal time:* you must eat single-handed at first, using only your unoperated arm. A "splade" (combined knife/fork/spoon) is extremely useful.

Domestic chores

◆ **Do not push or pull or lift with your operated arm in the first 6 weeks** (unless your surgery has been a simple arthroscopic acromioplasty).

◆ If you must do any *light* domestic household chores in the first 4 to 6 weeks, they must be done one-handed with your unoperated arm. Avoid all heavy household chores.

◆ Avoid lifting anything heavy for the first six weeks. After 4 weeks it is permissible to hold the equivalent of a cup of coffee in the hand of the operated arm, depending on advice from your surgeon. You will be weak at first, so go gently and carefully. Your therapist will guide you through the process of gradually increasing your day-to-day activities after the 6-week mark, but I have found that patients overdo this. Go slowly, both within your guidelines, and dependent on how the shoulder is feeling. If your shoulder gets a bit painful from overdoing your daily activities (after 6 weeks), don't panic, you haven't damaged anything. Simply ease off from your daily activities for a few days until the shoulder has settled—local heat or ice can help settle this increased soreness.

Posture and sit to stand

◆ Do not allow your operated shoulder to hunch up or be held forward. Sit and stand up straight, shoulders back and held at the same height.

◆ Do not pull your operated arm in the sling across the front of your body as this pulls the shoulder forward, leading to tightness in muscles and ligaments across the front of the shoulder.

◆ When rising from a chair, use your unaffected arm to help slide you forward to the edge of the seat. From this position you can push up with your legs and unaffected arm. Under no circumstances push up with your operated arm in the first 6 weeks. To sit, reverse the procedure - sit on the edge of the seat, then use your unaffected arm to help slide back into the chair.

Driving

◆ Do not drive while still wearing the sling. The surgeon will give you some guidelines, but even once out of the sling your pain and mobility of the shoulder must allow normal handling of steering and controls before resuming driving.

◆ As a passenger, it's important to protect the operated shoulder as you get in and out of the car. To get into the car, face away from the car and lower yourself down to the seat, using the strength of your legs with the help of your unaffected arm, before swinging your legs into the car. Reverse this for exiting the car. Ask for assistance from the driver if needed—don't be too proud to ask for help!

Sleeping

◆ If sleeping in a bed proves too difficult in the first couple of weeks, you may prefer to sleep semi-reclining in a reclining armchair. Your operated arm can be supported by pillows for comfort and the most pain free position.

◆ In bed you may get comfortable semi-reclining with pillows or a purpose made semi-reclining pillow or foam block. Reclining at 40° or less is recommended for best sleep.

◆ As your shoulder pain settles, you may be able to get comfortable lying flatter and even on your unaffected side using a pillow in front of you to support the operated arm.

Managing stairs

Always use a balustrade with the unaffected arm for balance and support while still using a sling.

Return to work

This is often the question first asked by patients when surgery is discussed. Your surgeon will advise. The time before returning to work will depend on many factors:

◆ The nature of your work. If you have a sedentary office job not involving physical tasks, you can probably resume work as soon as the pain settles and you feel able to eg after 2 to 3 weeks. If your work involves heavy manual tasks or lifting, you may need to wait 6 to 10 weeks to allow time for healing and strengthening.

◆ The type of procedure. With a simple arthroscopic acromioplasty, it will depend on how quickly the pain settles over the first 2 to 3 weeks. On the other hand, a rotator cuff repair or total shoulder replacement will require much longer for healing to take place, and you will need to wear a sling for up to 6 weeks. You will be restricted from using the arm for all but the simplest exercises in that time, so there will be a rehabilitation period of several weeks once you are out of the sling.

◆ How well you follow the advice from your surgeon, therapist and this book.

Chapter 13

Exercise - There Is No Other Option!

EVERY SHOULDER IS DIFFERENT...

For each type of shoulder surgery, and for each individual patient, the exercise rehabilitation program will be best designed by the orthopaedic surgeon and physiotherapist working together for the best outcome.

However, there are basic principles that apply to all shoulder surgery and all individuals. In this chapter I want to bring you to an understanding of these principles, so that you can steer confidently and intelligently through the complexities of your rehabilitation exercise program. I will explain the 4 phases of your recovery, give you sample exercises for each phase, and then explain how the progression through these phases differs with common types of shoulder surgery.

Let me explain my personal philosophy of postoperative shoulder rehabilitation. You will understand by now having read this far through this book, that you will experience some post-operative pain. In the immediate post-operative period, you will need to do some movements that may cause some temporary increase in shoulder pain. The mistakes that people make during the post-operative recovery fall into two categories:

◆ Those who are apprehensive and loath to cause any shoulder discomfort at all, holding their arm rigidly to their side in the sling. These patients are likely to have increased muscle tension in the neck, upper trapezius and upper back causing increased discomfort in these areas. They are also likely to be much slower to regain both passive and later active range of movement.

◆ On the other hand, there are those who do their exercises too enthusiastically or too aggressively. In this group patients are often prone to ignore specific instructions from the surgeon to limit certain movements of the shoulder. These patients are likely to experience at some point during their rehabilitation periods of marked increase in shoulder pain, which slows their progress. Ignoring the specific instructions of the surgeon can also cause failure of the repaired structures in the shoulder.

So my philosophy for rehabilitation of the shoulder is basically this: move the shoulder gently but frequently in the early stages of recovery, always remembering the specific limitations placed on your movements by the surgeon. As you progress through the rehabilitation exercise program, you should not be causing pain with any particular exercise. If you experience pain, you need to modify your exercise technique, or decrease the resistance or number of repetitions, or both. If you have inadvertently caused your shoulder to become quite sore after exercise, use ice or heat to settle the pain. Do not push your exercises as hard at the next session—in fact don't hesitate to leave your exercises for the rest of that day.

One other point—don't be tempted to stop your rehab exercises once the shoulder is pain free. If you want to return to full range of movement and function (and stay that way), you need to persevere with your rehabilitation exercise program.

PHASES OF RECOVERY

Phase 1: Protect the Joint / Early Movement

◆ This phase lasts 1 to 6 weeks, depending on the type of surgery.

◆ The goals are to protect the healing tissues in the shoulder, maintain mobility with gentle passive movements, activate muscles in the scapula area, prevent muscle inhibition, and maintain movement in elbow, wrist & fingers.

◆ During this phase movements are done *passively* by your other arm or by the therapist. During passive movements there is no contraction of the shoulder muscles. It is critical to keep stresses off healing structures, especially for rotator cuff repairs.

◆ On the other hand, you can actively move the elbow, wrist and fingers as long as the shoulder is protected.

◆ The scapular muscles can also be activated without putting stress on the healing shoulder.

Phase 2: Active-Assisted to Active Movement Phase

◆ Weeks 6 to 10.

◆ You will start to activate the shoulder muscles, while assisting the movement with gravity or your other arm. These "active-assisted" exercises gradually progress to fully "active" exercises as the post-operative healing progresses.

◆ The goal is to restore full passive range of motion while still not over-stressing the healing tissues. This is a stage where patients often become over enthusiastic about their exercises, leading to increased shoulder pain and potentially poorer healing.

Phase 3: Early Strengthening Phase

◆ Weeks 10 to 16.

◆ The goals progress now—you will still work to improve and maintain your range of shoulder movement, but active strengthening against the resistance of bands, weights and gravity becomes important.

◆ During this period you will work on the gradual restoration of shoulder strength, power, endurance and dynamic stability.

◆ There will also be a gradual return to functional activities.

Phase 4: Advanced Strengthening Phase

◆ Week 16 onwards.

◆ The goal now is to maintain your range of movement while progressing your strengthening program. This will allow you to return to your ultimate functional activities without risk of injury to the shoulder.

◆ During this phase you can begin a "return to sport" progressive program, which includes exercises specific to the sport you wish to return to.

EXERCISES FOR EACH PHASE

Phase 1: Protect the Joint / Early Movement

Hand gripping (in the sling): squeeze and release a soft ball repeatedly throughout the day. This exercise maintains your grip strength, but more importantly tightening the muscles of the forearm helps pump fluid out of your arm, preventing your resting arm from swelling.

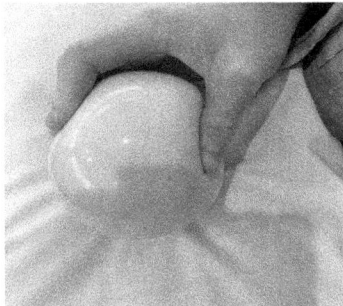

Elbow bend/straighten: release your forearm from the sling. If sitting or standing stabilize your upper arm with your other hand. If lying, rest your elbow on a pillow. Straighten your elbow as far as possible and bend as far as possible. Repeat x10.

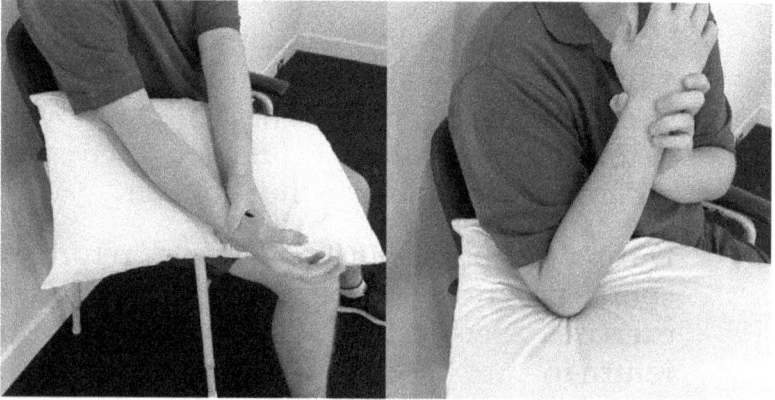

Finger, wrist and forearm range of motion exercises: Make a fist, then stretch your fingers and thumb out straight. Whilst still in the sling, bend your wrist back and forth, then rotate the forearm fully one way and back the other way. Repeat x10 for each movement.

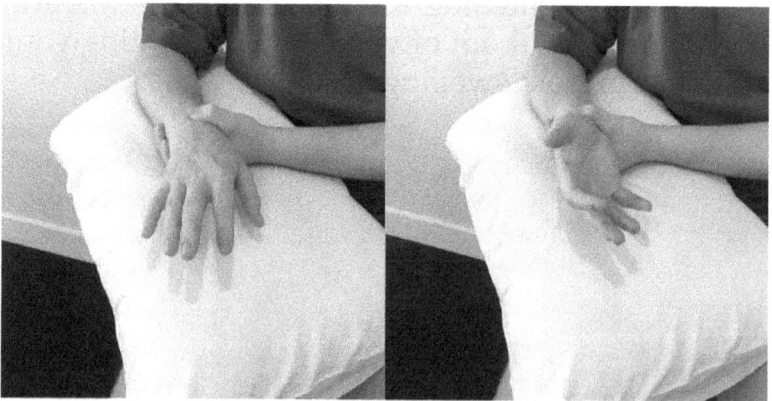

Neck range of motion:

Turn your head to look fully over your left shoulder, then back to look over your right shoulder. Repeat×10.

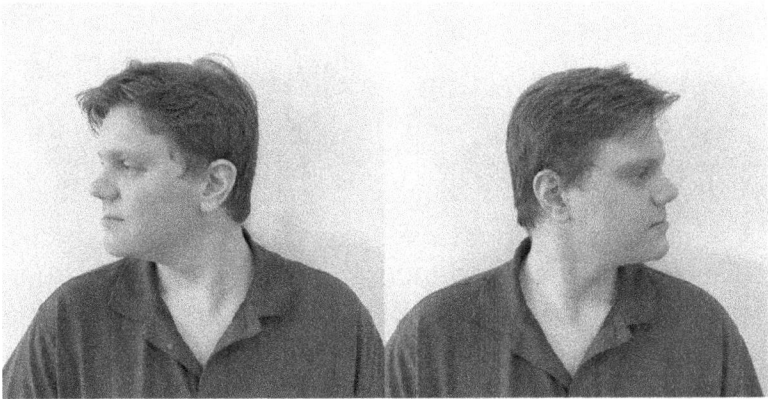

Tilt your head over to the left taking your ear towards the tip of your shoulder, then reverse to tilt towards the right shoulder. Repeat x10.

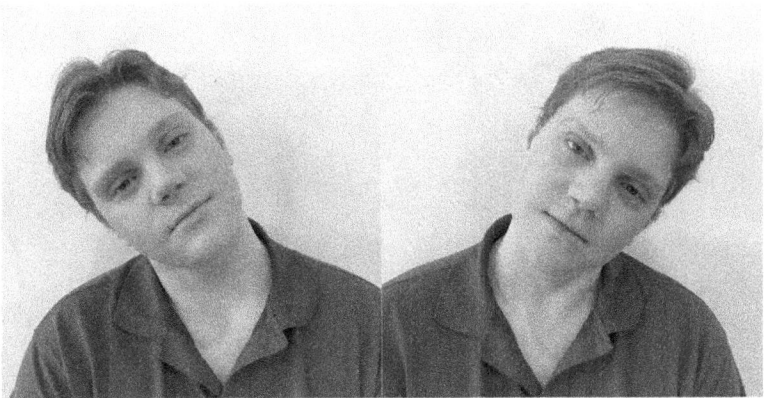

Shoulder blade (scapula) movements: Sitting with your arms by your side pull your shoulder blades back and down, squeezing them towards each other. Hold for five seconds, then relax. Repeat x10.

97

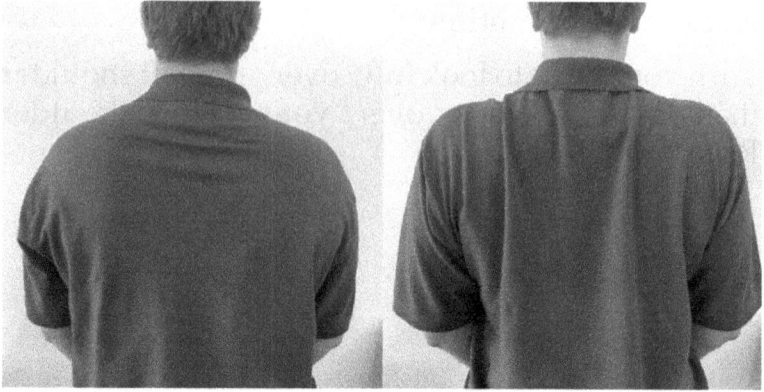

"Chin tucks" posture exercise: This exercise counteracts the tendency that we all have when sitting of adopting a "chin forward" posture. Sitting up straight in a chair against a backrest, pull your neck and upper back up straight by gliding your head backwards. Your face should remain vertical, and you should have the feeling of creating "double chins." Hold for five seconds. Repeat x10.

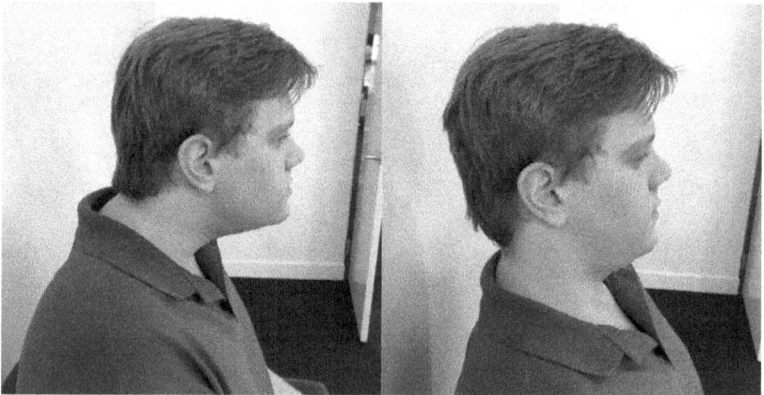

Passive range of motion exercises:

Rock-a-bye cradle pendulums: Bend forward at the waist and use your good arm to support the forearm and elbow of the operated arm. Use your good arm to move the elbow in small circles x10 each direction, then move the operated arm back and forwards x10. As each week goes by make the circles and the swing back and forwards gradually bigger and bend further forward at the waist.

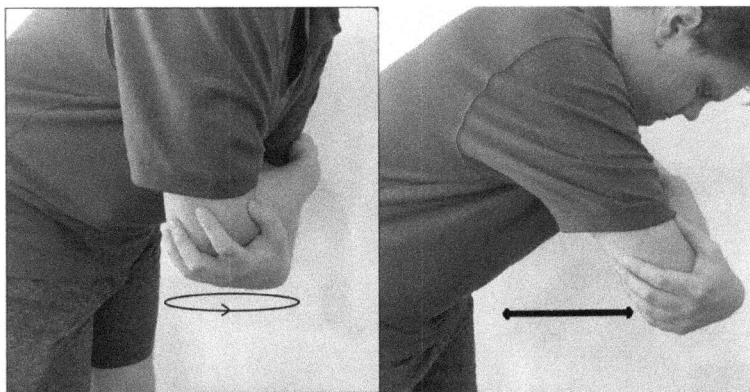

Pendular exercises: Bend forward, supporting your weight on your unaffected arm. Keeping your spine straight, let your operated arm hang relaxed straight down and swing in small circles, x10 in each direction. Start this movement by using small movements of your upper body to get the arm swinging. Also swing the arm gently back and forth by your side, x10.

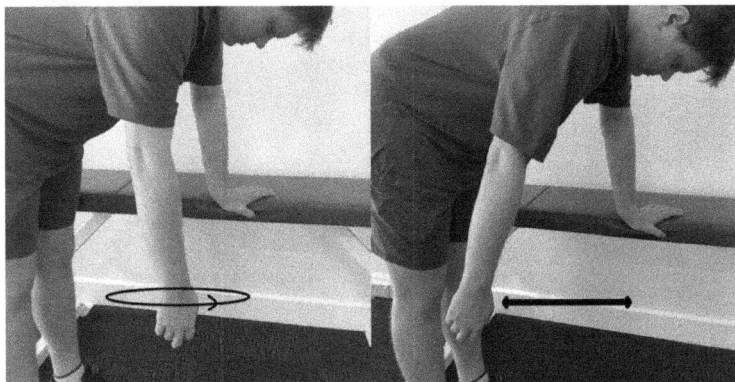

Passive flexion table stretch: Place your palms on the top of a table or bench and step back gently, bending at the waist until you feel a gentle stretch around the shoulder. Hold the stretch for five seconds, repeat x10.

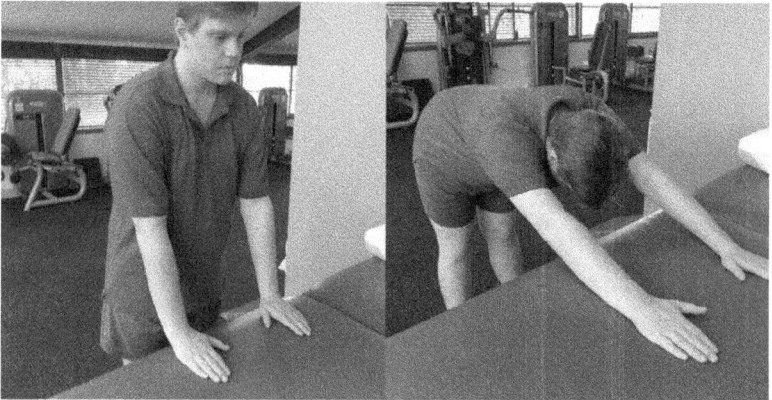

Passive external rotation (seated or supine): With the arm supported and the elbow bent to 90°, reach across with the unaffected arm and gently rotate the operated arm out to the side just to the point of tightness, not pain. Hold the stretch for five seconds, repeat x10.

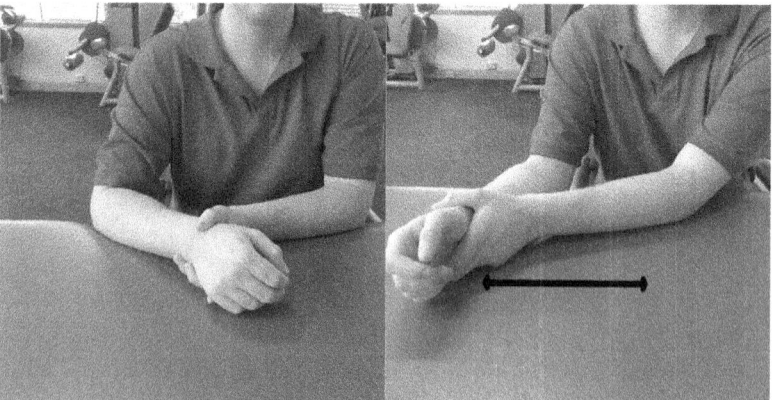

Walking or stationary bike: From Week 2 onwards you can start a few minutes every day on a stationary bike or walking to improve and maintain cardiovascular fitness.

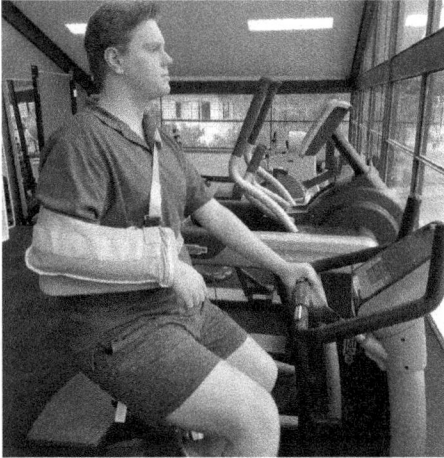

Phase 2: Active-Assisted to Active Movement

Auto-assisted flexion lying with stick: Lying on your back, hold a short length of broomstick hands close together. Raise the stick and arms up and over as far as possible with the unaffected arm helping the operated arm. Repeat x5, build up to x10.

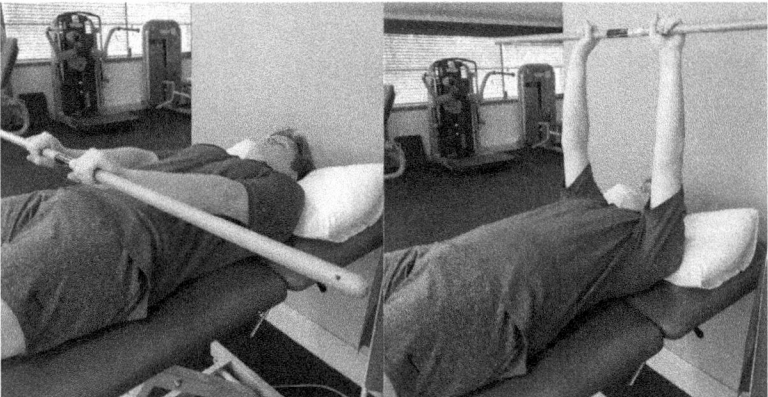

External rotation with stick: Hold the broomstick with both hands shoulder width apart and with the elbows bent to 90°. Use the unaffected arm to push the hand of the operated arm out to the side until you feel tightness. Keep the elbow tucked into the side. Hold for five seconds. Repeat x10.

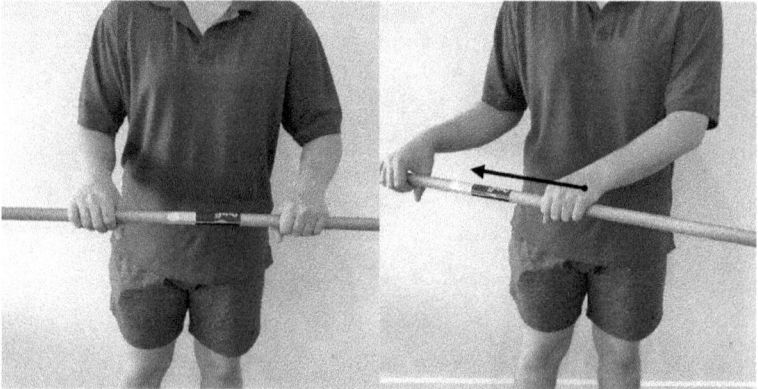

Overhead pulley for flexion: Attach a pulley to the wall or the top of a door. Stand facing the door and pull down with your unaffected arm to gently stretch the operated arm as high as possible. Hold for five seconds, then relax. Repeat x10.

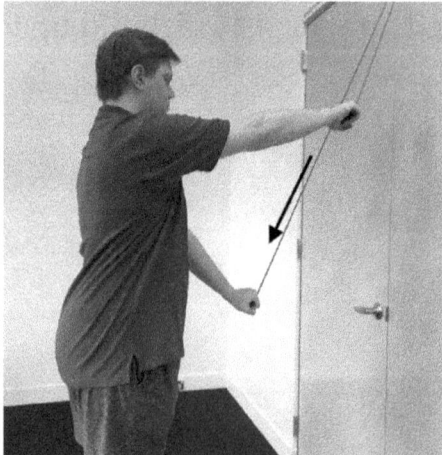

Overhead pulley for abduction: Stand with the operated arm towards the door and pull down with your unaffected arm to gently stretch the operated arm as high as possible up to the side. Hold for five seconds, then relax. Repeat x10.

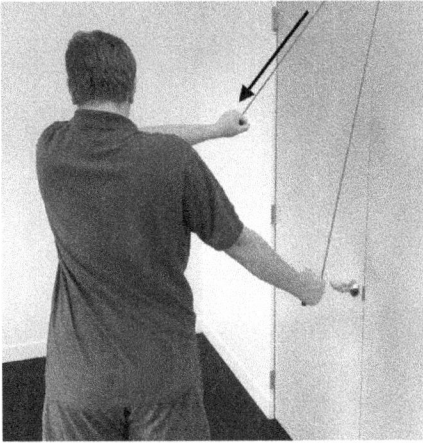

Lying alphabet writing: Lying on your back raise the operated arm to vertical assisted by the unaffected arm. Describe the letters of the alphabet in the air—small letters at first, getting bigger over repeated sessions.

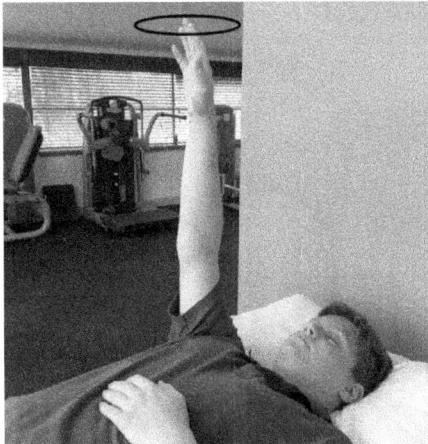

Auto-assisted walk fingers up wall—flexion: Face the wall, and assist your operated arm with your unaffected arm by supporting under the elbow. Walk your fingertips up the wall until you feel a gentle stretch. Assist your arm to slide your fingers down the wall. Repeat x5.

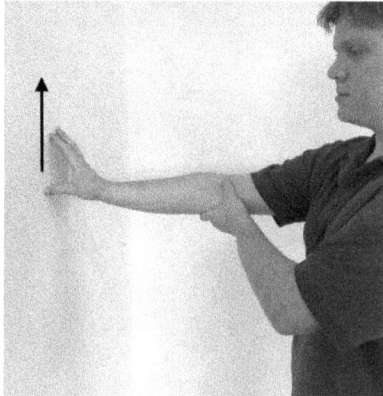

Phase 3: Early Strengthening Phase

Walk fingers up wall—flexion and abduction: Both facing the wall and side on to the wall, walk your fingers up the wall as far as possible until you feel the stretch. Hold 5 seconds, then slide your fingers back down the wall. Repeat x10.

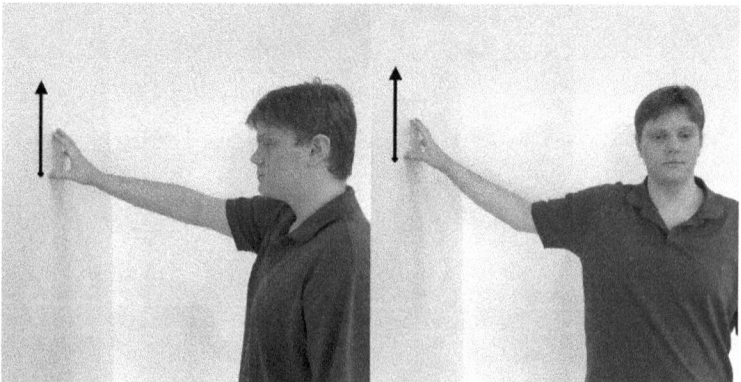

Begin early hand behind back stretch: Reach across behind your back with your unaffected arm. Grasp the hand of the operated arm and draw towards the middle of your back *until you feel a gentle stretch but no pain.* Hold 5 seconds, repeat x5.

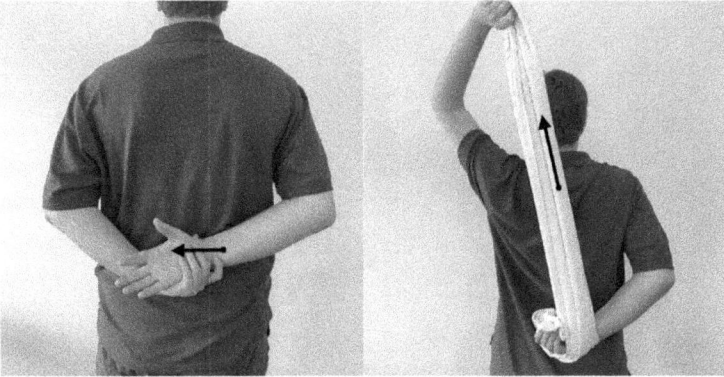

You can extend this exercise over time by using a towel to draw the hand of your operated arm up the centre of your back. *You must do this exercise gently.*

Stretch posterior shoulder capsule: Draw your arm across your body with the other hand on your elbow. Hold for 10 seconds, repeat x3.

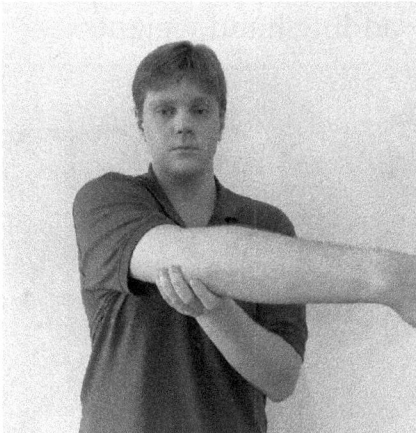

Roll ball on wall: stand facing the wall with your hand holding a small ball against the wall. Roll the ball in circles on the wall, ensuring that your shoulder blade is held back and down. Continue for 1 minute, repeat x2.

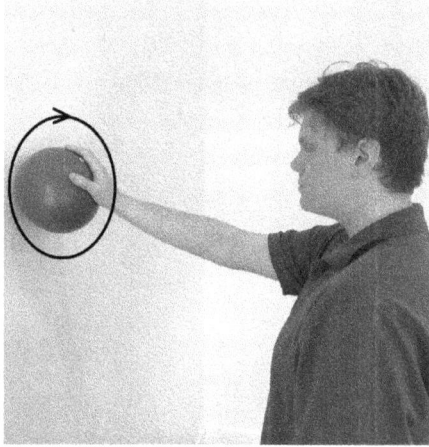

Lying push hand to ceiling: Lying on your back, raise your straight arm to vertical. Slowly push up towards the ceiling raising your shoulder blade off the surface, hold 5 seconds then slowly lower the shoulder blade to the surface. Repeat x10. Progress over time by adding hand weights.

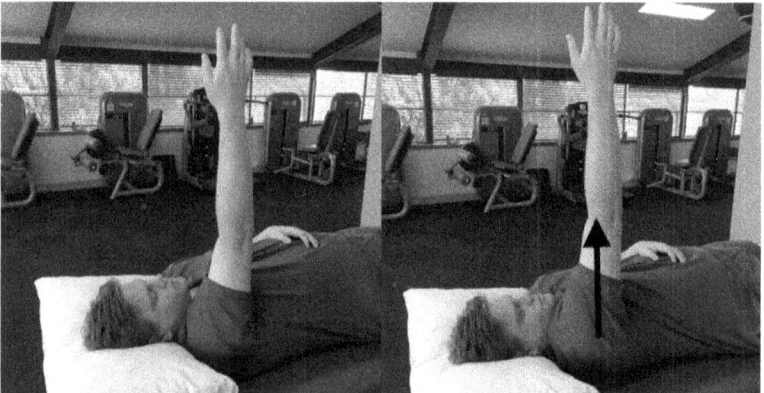

Exercises with bands (start with red band)

Elbow Straight:

Pull down from front: Attach the band to a point at shoulder height and face the band attachment. Keeping the arm straight, pull *slowly* down to the side of your leg, pause, then resist the band as your arm *slowly* returns to the start position. Repeat x10.

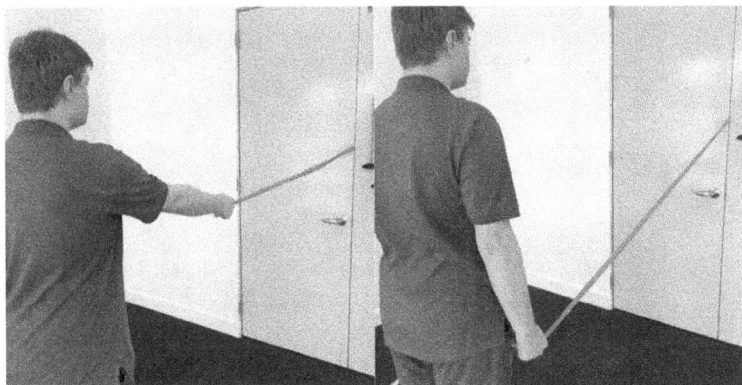

Pull down from side: Stand side on to the attachment point. Keeping the arm straight, pull *slowly* down to the side of your leg, pause, then resist the band as your arm *slowly* returns to your starting position. Repeat x10.

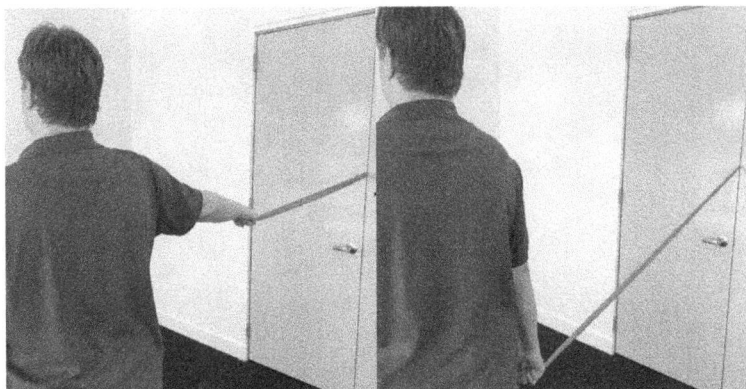

Pull forward from behind: Attach the band to a point at waist height and face away from the band attachment point. Keep the arm straight, pull *slowly* forward, pause, then resist the band as your arm *slowly* returns to your starting position. Repeat x10.

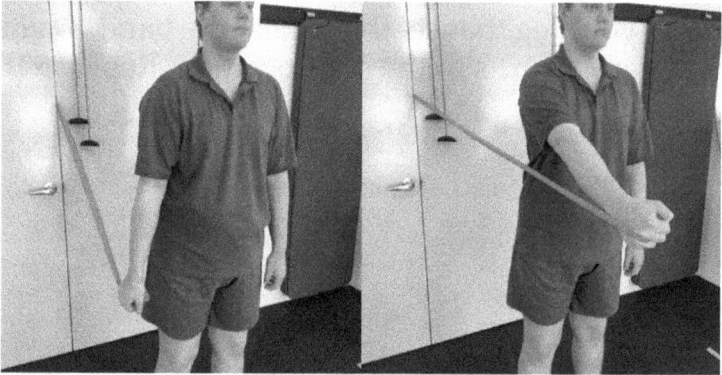

Elbow Bent:

Pull in across abdomen: Attach the band to a point at waist height and stand with the operated arm towards the band attachment point. Keeping the elbow bent to 90° and the shoulder blades held back, pull slowly inwards across the body, pause, then resist the band as your arm slowly returns to your starting position. Repeat x10.

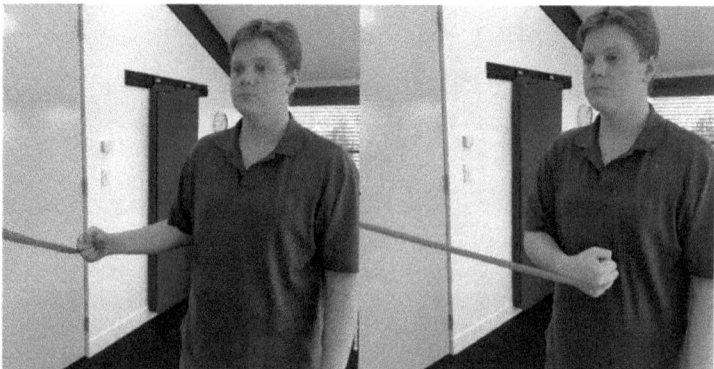

Pull out from across abdomen: Stand with the operated arm away from the band attachment point. Keeping the elbow bent to 90° and the shoulder blades held back, pull slowly outwards from across the body as far as you can *comfortably*, pause, then resist the band as your arm slowly returns to your starting position. Repeat x10.

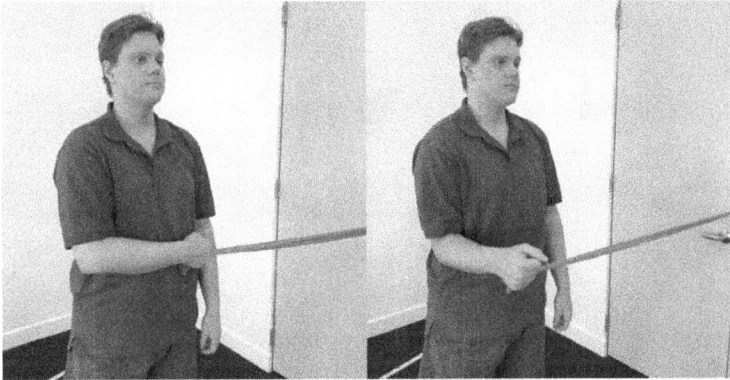

Single arm row: Face towards the band attachment point. Keeping the shoulder blades held back, start with the arm outstretched, slowly bend the elbow, pulling the band into the body, with the elbow going the past the waist, pause, then resist the band as your arm slowly returns. Repeat x10.

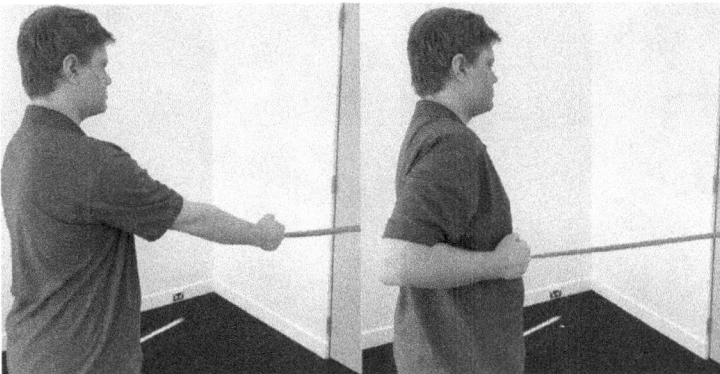

Biceps curl: Stand on one end of the band and hold the other end with your arm by your side. Slowly bend your elbow as far as you can, pause, then resist the band as your arm slowly returns to your starting position. Repeat x10.

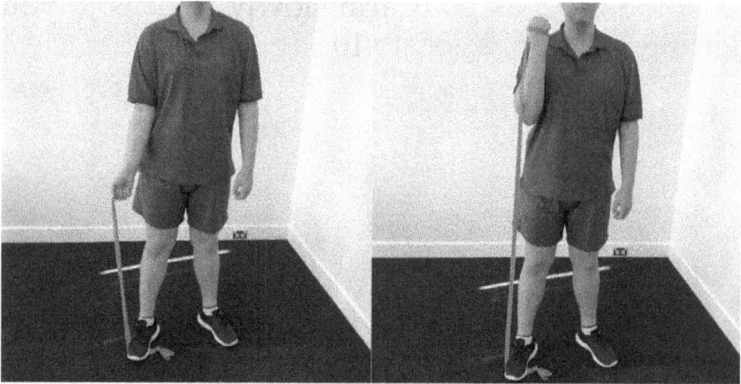

Triceps extension: Attach the band at shoulder height, stand facing towards the attachment point. Start with the elbow bent to 90° and the shoulder blades held back. Pull slowly down to your side as you straighten the elbow, pause, then resist the band as your arm slowly returns to your starting position. Repeat x10.

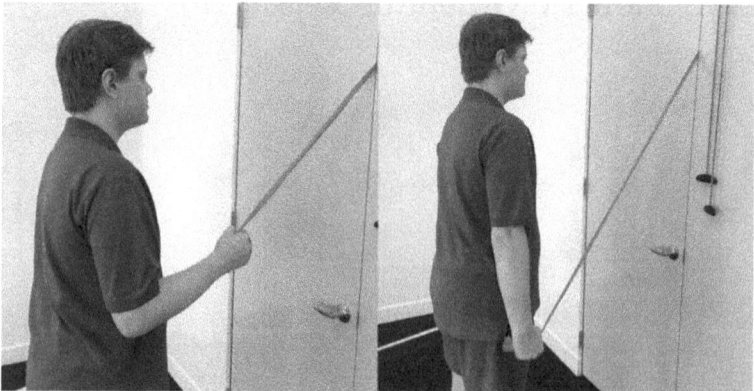

Wall push-offs: Stand facing towards the wall. Place your hands against the wall with straight elbows. The movement is a pushing away from the wall using only the movement of your shoulder blades as you push them forward, hold, then slowly pull the shoulder blades back and down as your body moves towards the wall. These are small controlled slow movements. Repeat x10.

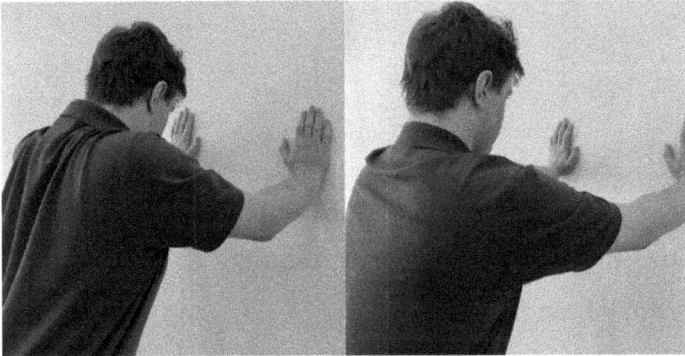

Standing alphabet: Stand with your back against the wall and your arm held out horizontally with your shoulder blades set back. Describe the letters of the alphabet in the air—small letters at first, getting bigger over repeated sessions.

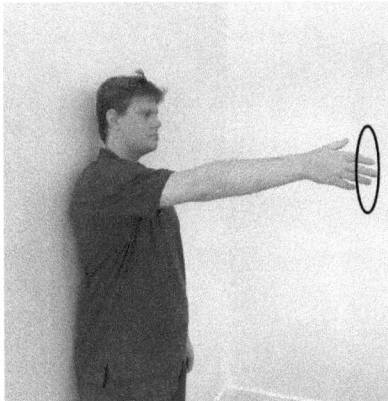

Overhead hands clap: Starting with your arms by your side, set your shoulder blades back and raise your arms into an overhead clap. Repeat x10.

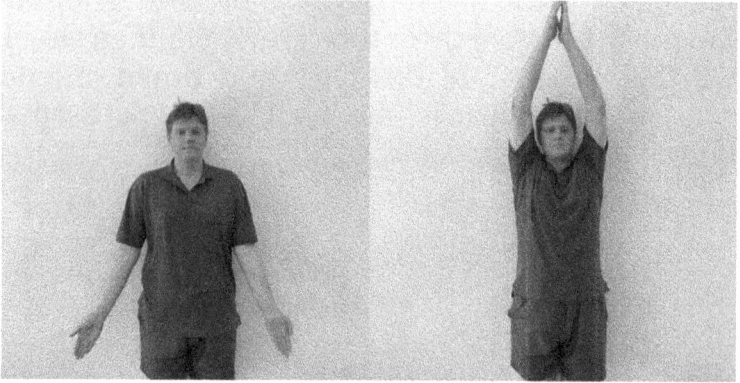

Phase 4: Advanced Strengthening & Stretching

Strengthening:

Bent over scapula row: Start in a bent over, supported position with the spine straight and your operated arm hanging towards the floor with a hand weight (start with 0.5kg). Slowly pull the shoulder blade back lifting the weight with the arm kept straight, pause and lower slowly. Repeat x10.

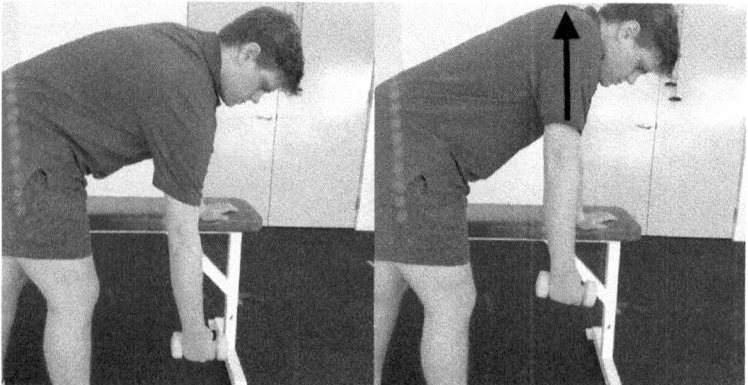

Prone scapula retraction: Lie face down with the head supported, the arms by the side resting on the surface. Slowly lift the shoulders off the surface, squeezing the shoulder blades towards each other. Hold for 5 seconds, then slowly relax. Repeat x10. Shoulders should not hitch up, neck stays relaxed.

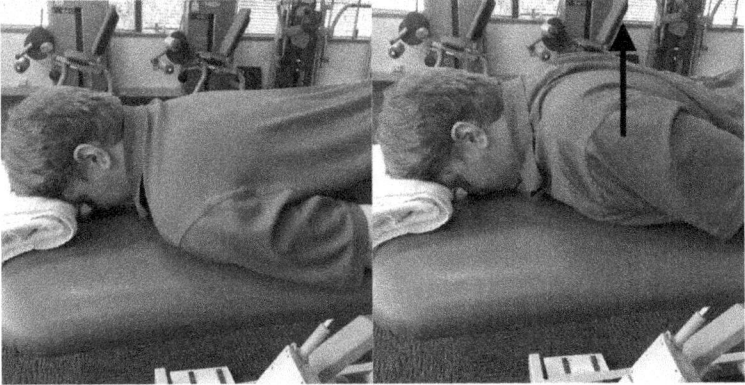

To increase the difficulty over time, once the shoulder blades have been lifted, then raise the arms off the surface.

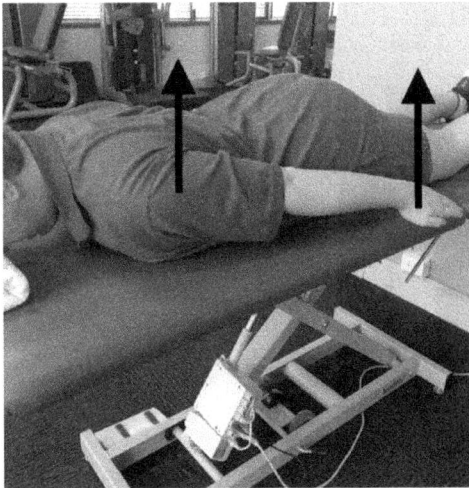

Prone arm lifts: A more advanced exercise than the "prone scapula retraction." Start with the same lift off the surface with the arm, then slowly move the arm around to above the head, pause, then slowly return to the starting position and relax. Repeat x10.

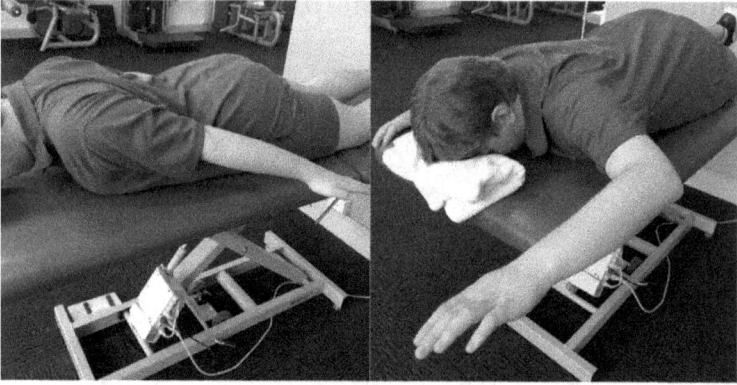

Overhead triceps extension: Support your arm with the unaffected arm in the overhead position as shown, holding a small hand weight (start with 1kg). Slowly lower the weight behind your shoulder, then raise it smoothly until the elbow is fully extended. Repeat x10. Keep your neck and upper trapezius relaxed.

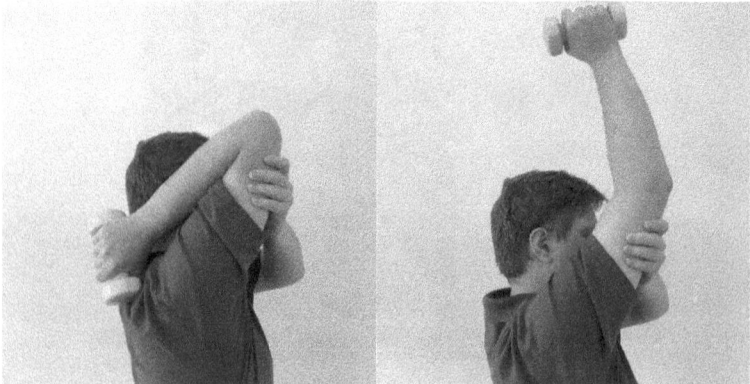

Serratus punch forward: Attach the band to a point at shoulder height. Start by standing with your opposite foot forward and the end of the band in your hand, shoulder blade retracted as shown. Slowly push the band forward while rotating the trunk forward. Hold 5 seconds, slowly return.

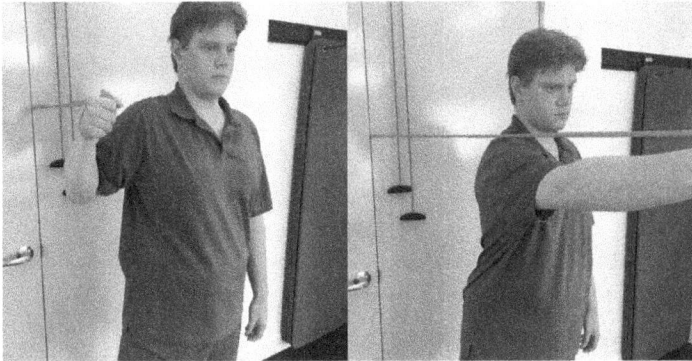

Scapula push-offs: Stand with your hands against the wall, straight elbows, lean into wall, body held straight. Push away from the wall using only the movement of your shoulder blades as you push them forward, hold, then slowly pull the shoulder blades back and down as your body moves towards the wall. Note that these are small controlled slow movements. Repeat x10.

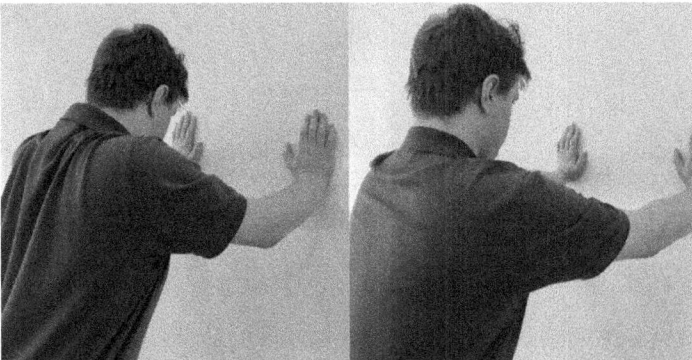

To extend difficulty, stand further away from the wall, then progress to working off the edge of a bench.

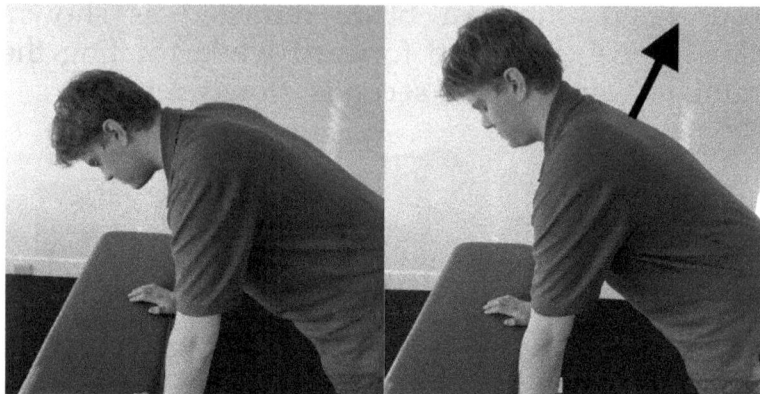

External rotation in abduction: Attach the band at shoulder height. Stand facing the band with the elbow bent to 90° and the arm raised away from the side (45° at first, progressing later to 90°). Pull back slowly with your hand, maintaining the same angle of your arm away from your body, pause, then slowly return to the starting position. Repeat x10. Keep the shoulder blade depressed, and the neck relaxed.

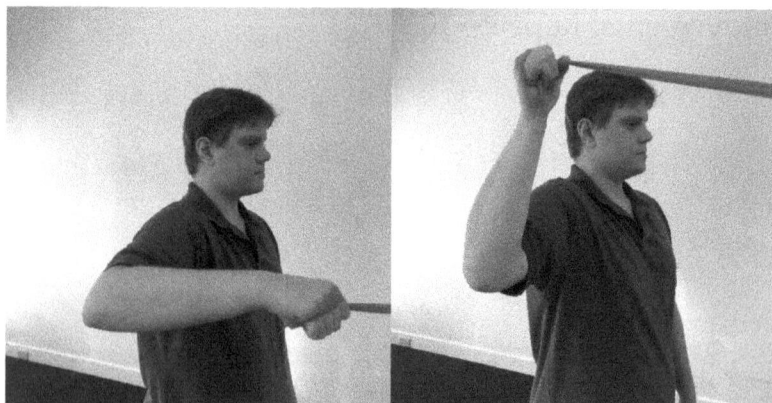

Internal rotation in abduction: Stand facing away from the band with the elbow bent to 90° and the arm raised away from the side (45° at first, progressing later to 90°). Pull forward slowly with your hand, maintaining the same angle of your arm away from your body, pause, then slowly return. Repeat x10.

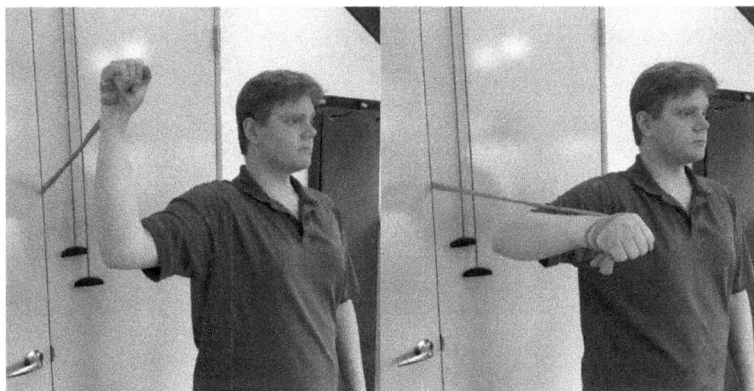

Diagonal pull with band—inside to outside: Stand with the band in your hand and the band under your foot on the opposite side. Starting with your arm slightly across your body, pull the band up and across your body to a stop sign position. Repeat x 10. Build up to 3 sets.

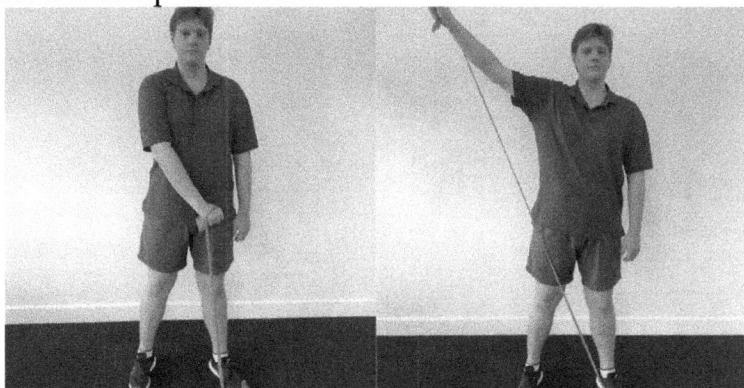

Diagonal pull with band—outside to inside: Stand with the band in your hand and the band under your foot on the same side. Pull the band up and across your body as far as possible. Repeat x 10. Build up to 3 sets.

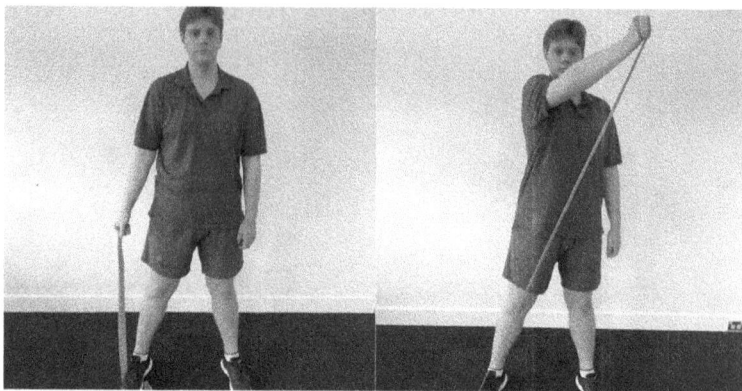

Stretching:

Overhead stretch: Grasp an overhead bar, hands shoulder width apart. Lower your weight slightly to gently stretch both shoulders Hold for 10 seconds repeat x3.

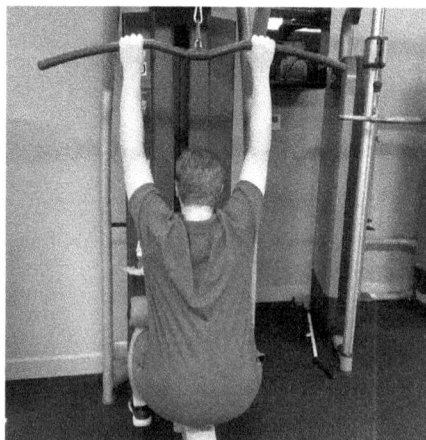

Trunk (thoracic) rotation: With arms folded across your chest, twist the upper body to each side. Hold for 5 seconds at each side, repeat x3.

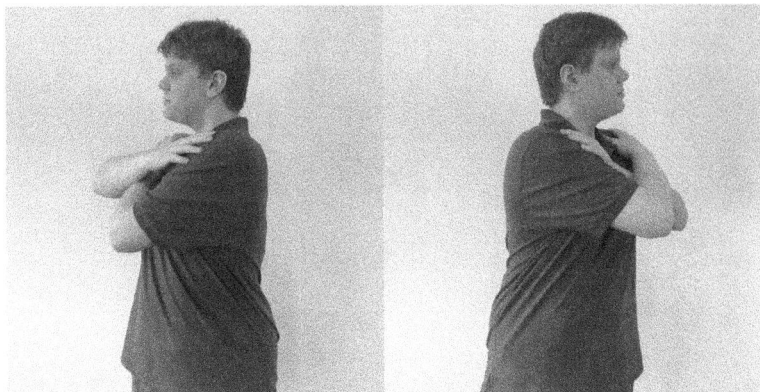

Posterior deltoid/shoulder capsule: Draw your arm across your body with the other hand on your elbow until you feel a gentle stretch. Hold for 10 seconds, repeat x3.

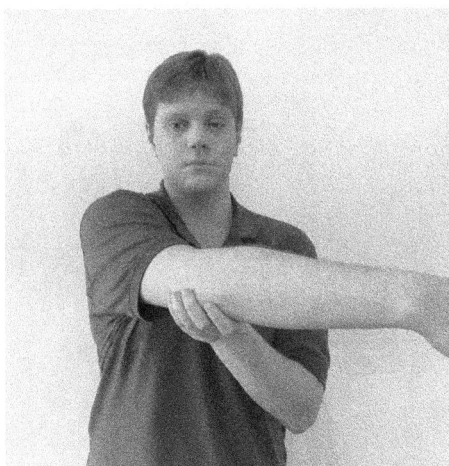

Triceps: Raise your arm forward to the limit, then drop your hand down your back. Grasp your elbow with your other hand and stretch up and over. Hold for 10 seconds, repeat x3.

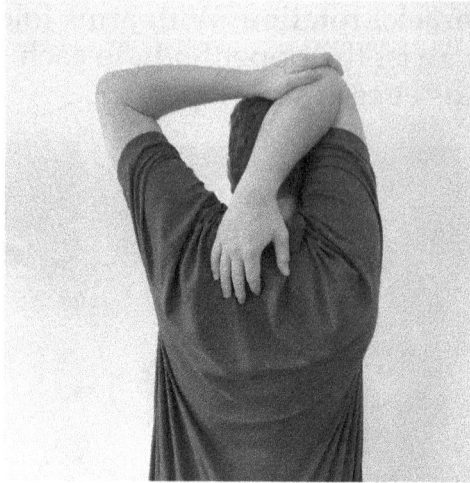

Rhomboids: Interlock your fingers and push your palms forward, stretching the muscles across your upper back. Hold for 10 seconds, repeat x3.

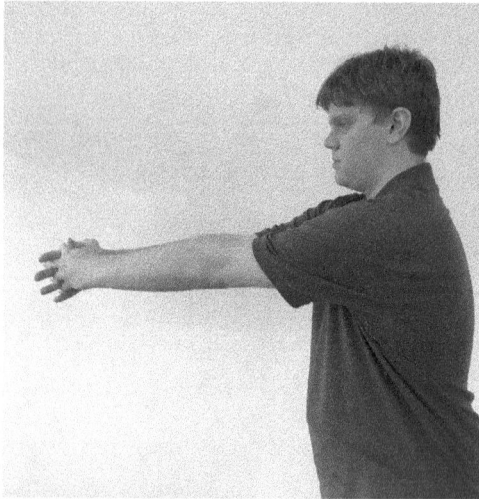

Lower pectorals: Interlock your fingers and push your hands out behind you, stretching the muscles across the front of your chest. Hold for 10 seconds, repeat x3.

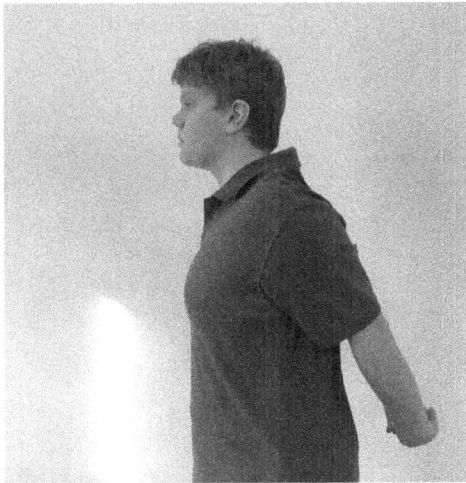

Stop sign: Place your arm against a door frame in a stop position—turn your body away slightly until you feel a gentle stretch across your chest and shoulder. Hold for 10 seconds, repeat x3.

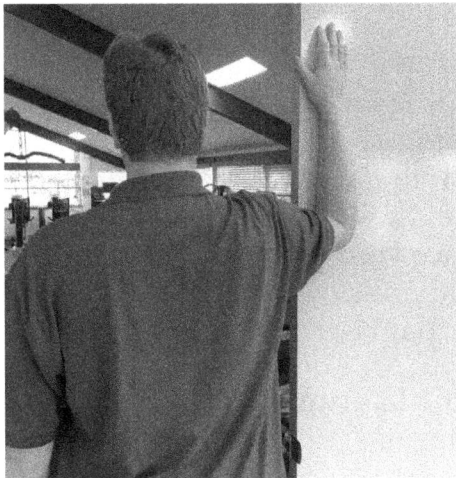

External rotation: Place your hand against a doorframe and hold the elbow against your side with the other hand. Stretch the arm outwards by turning your body away until you feel a *gentle*

stretch. Hold for 10 seconds, repeat x3.

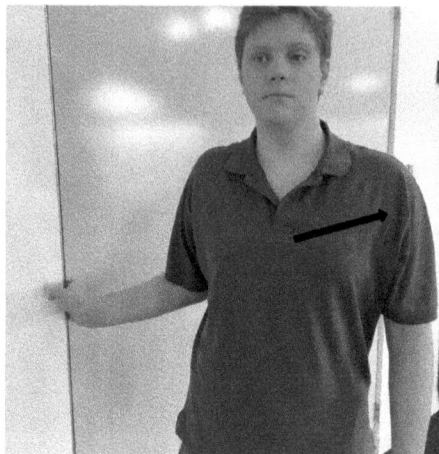

SPECIFIC ADVICE FOR YOUR SURGERY

Arthroscopic Acromioplasty/Subacromial Decompression

While you will wear a sling when you leave hospital, this is for comfort and to settle the pain in the immediate post-operative days. You will be encouraged to move the shoulder fairly quickly through the phases of recovery, and dispense with the sling once your pain has settled sufficiently. Use ice frequently and you should see a rapid decrease in shoulder pain over the first two weeks.

Arthroscopic Labrum Repair & Shoulder Stabilization

The whole purpose of this surgery is to stabilise the shoulder, so we are more concerned that you protect the healing tissues from being over-stressed. Follow your surgeon's advice about restrictions of movement conscientiously. You will be in a sling for at least 4 weeks and during this time you will not actively exercise against any resistance, not even the weight of the arm. You may not drive during the time you're still in the sling.

Acromioclavicular Joint Stabilization

Again, the whole purpose of this surgery is to stabilise the ACJ, so we are concerned that you protect the healing tissues from being over-stressed. Follow your surgeon's advice about restrictions of movement conscientiously. You will be in a sling for at least 4 weeks and during this time you may not drive.

Rotator Cuff Repair

For a rotator cuff repair, it's important to remember that even at six weeks when you come out of the sling the rotator cuff repair is probably only a fraction of its ultimate strength. So when you enter Phase 2 at six weeks post-operative, your repair is still fragile, and during Phase 2 you'll be doing active *assisted* exercises. Having said that, it's still important to move the shoulder regularly to improve and maintain your range of movement.

Total Shoulder Replacement

Although the components of your new shoulder joint are quite stable immediately after surgery, there are other tissues that require time to heal. One of your rotator cuff tendons—the subscapularis— has been separated from the bone to allow access and then reattached. Also, the biceps tendon has probably been re-attached to the upper humerus. With this in mind you will need to wear a sling for about four weeks and there will be specific instructions about not pushing the shoulder into external rotation past a certain number of degrees (e.g. 30°) and not actively internally rotating against any resistance.

So a last but important piece of advice: *follow your surgeon's instructions about what movements to avoid and when to start moving the shoulder.* Your surgeon knows the details of what techniques were used during your surgery and thus what *your* specific restrictions are.

Chapter 14

Return to Work, Sport & Recreation

The timing of your return to work, sport (either social or competitive) and recreational activities will vary from person-to-person depending on:

♦ The type and scope of your work, sport and recreation.

♦ The type of surgery you have undergone.

♦ The extent of the repair and changes to the structure of the shoulder for your particular surgery.

♦ The time you have been absent from these activities, and accordingly the degree of your loss of fitness specific to that activity.

Before you attempt to return to work, sport and recreational activities you should be assessed by a physiotherapist. They will advise on which activities you are fit enough for, and which activities will demand you wait until your strength or range of movement has improved further.

Work

If you have a desk job, then your return to work duties will be typically much faster–you may be ready to return to work 6 to 8 weeks after rotator cuff repair, for instance. If you're able to work with one arm in the sling and out of action, then you can return to work even sooner. On the other hand, if you lift, push or pull at work, you will probably need between 3 to 6 months off work. In some cases, it may take up to 12 months before you can perform strenuous overhead activities.

Sport

The decision to return to sport will depend on what actions your sport requires, and at what level you play that sport. Your Physiotherapist will have modified your rehabilitation program, taking these factors into account. Your exercises will have been designed to give you the specific mobility, strength and endurance of your shoulder you need for your sport. Before even considering returning to competitive sport, regain a full range of movement in all directions and full strength of all shoulder movements.

Athletes undergoing many types of shoulder surgery may be advised that they should be capable of returning to their chosen sport six months postoperatively. Unfortunately this is often the case only in simpler types of shoulder surgery e.g. arthroscopic acromioplasty. In my experience, athletes who have had a rotator cuff repair need up to 12 months for unrestricted participation in contact or overhead sports.

Type of Surgery

Arthroscopic acromioplasty allows for a comparatively rapid recovery, with a sling being used for one to two weeks for comfort. You can progress your exercises at a pace dependent on your shoulder pain settling. You would expect to return to your regular work and sport after 2 to 4 months. The biggest fault I see in patients rehabilitating from arthroscopic acromioplasty is an overabundance of enthusiasm which can lead to a flareup of shoulder pain. Sensible progression through the range of exercises, applying ice after exercise if the shoulder gets sore, will see you make consistent progress.

Arthroscopic labrum repair / shoulder stabilization / acromioclavicular stabilisation surgeries will require you to allow enough time for healing, and for the stabilisation procedures to produce an effective result. Thus you will be in a sling for 4 to 6 weeks and participation in sports at any level won't start until after six months. I would urge you to progress gradually and aim for a return to normal sport (or demanding work) at 12 months postoperatively.

Rotator cuff repair requires you to protect the repair whilst still passively moving the shoulder. The strength of the repair improves slowly over 3 to 6 months, so your return to sport and work will depend on these activities and also on regaining full range of motion. The nature of your sport will influence your return:

◆ for bowls (considering the weight of the ball) expect 4 to 5 months,

- for golf 5 to 8 months,

- for resistance training at gym 6 to 12 months (with the resistance progressed slowly), and

- for contact and overhead sports 9 to 12 months.

Total shoulder replacement–it takes from 3 to 6 months for the shoulder to heal, and reaching your ultimate strength and range of motion can take 12 to 15 months. But most people find their shoulder pain has settled sufficiently to perform routine household and daily activities within three months. Depending on shoulder pain and mobility, you can expect to be driving by about 8 to 10 weeks. With the right exercises in your rehab program, sport like golf should be possible by six months. As you draw closer to returning to golf, include gentle golf swings in your exercise program.

Sports such as tennis are more problematic–if you have achieved an acceptable pain-free range of movement motion then you may return to some form of tennis (although surgeons warn that the shoulder replacement may wear more rapidly).

In summary, listen to your physiotherapist's advice, listen to what your shoulder is telling you, and don't push the limits! Make your return to sport and work a graduated return. Your shoulder will soon tell you if you're overdoing it. And importantly, make your exercise program specific to your particular work or sport.

Above all, don't hesitate to turn to a physiotherapist with a special interest in shoulders for advice during your recovery. Physiotherapists such as myself offer both face to face and telehealth online video consultations for shoulder rehabilitation.

You can also refer to my website www.theshoulderphysio.com for more information about managing your shoulder.

I wish you a speedy recovery from your shoulder surgery.

If you have found this book useful, to make the book more easily found by those who need it, I would be grateful if you could help with any of the following:

◆ Post a review on Amazon, Goodreads, your blog or any other website.
◆ Tell your friends or anyone you think would benefit from this book.
◆ Recommend or mention this book in any online forum or social media.
◆ Buy a copy for anyone who needs it!

Thank you.

Bruce Paulik, August 2020.